Family Planning and Reproductive Health

Edited by Zouhair Amarin and Hassan Abduljabbar

Published in London, United Kingdom

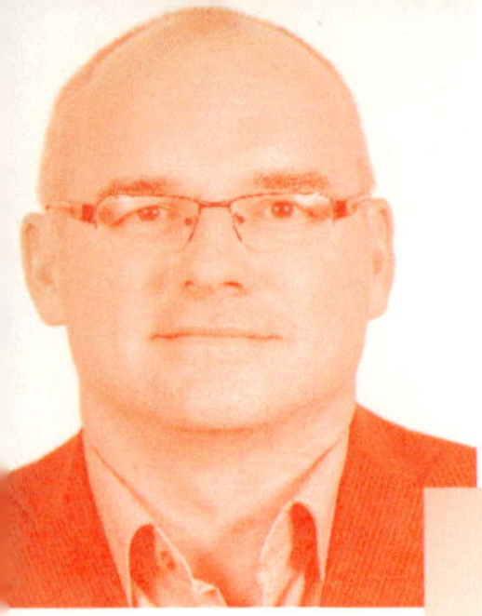
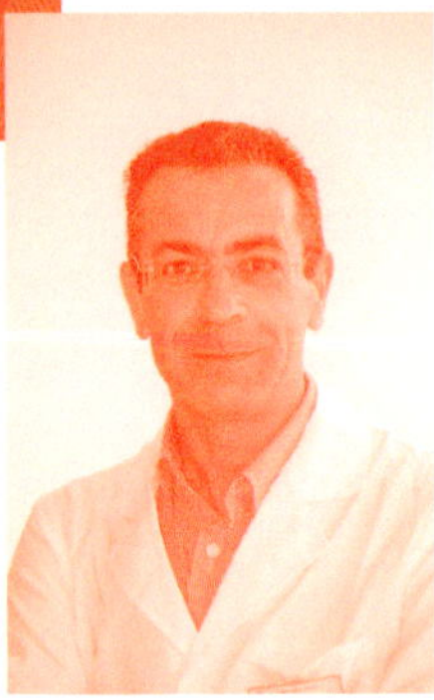
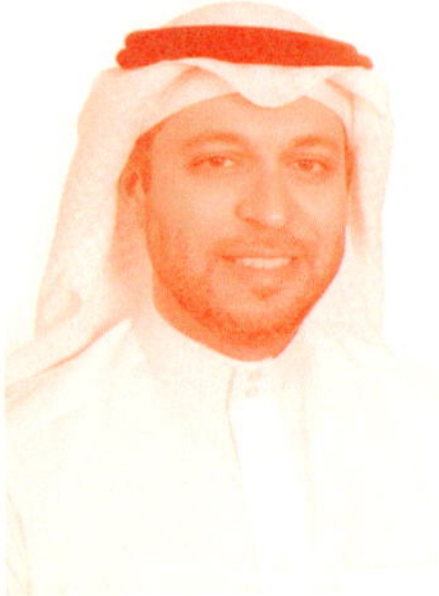
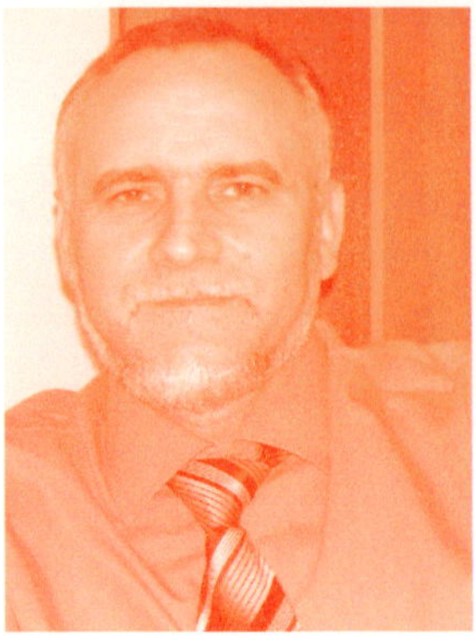
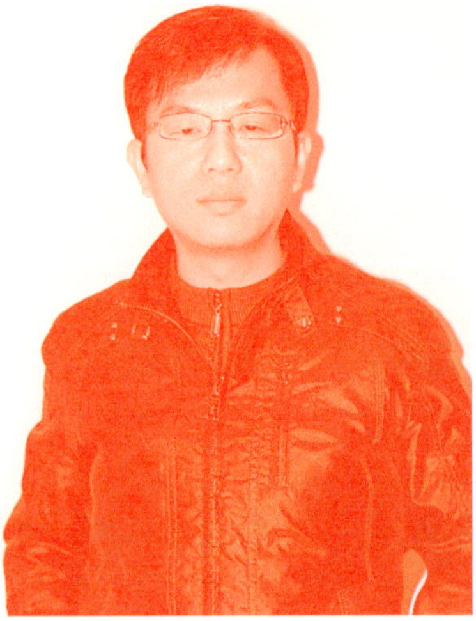
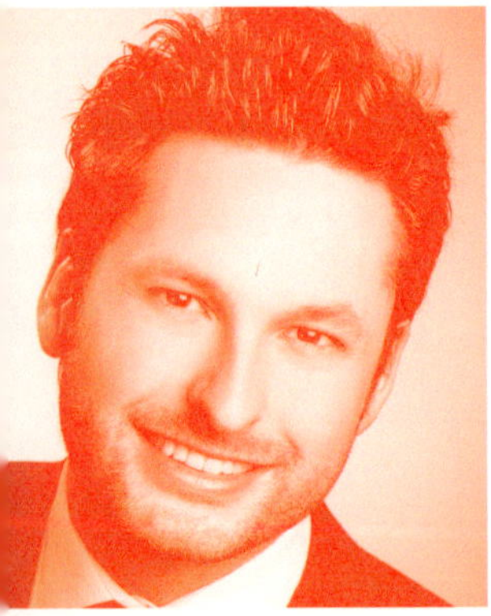
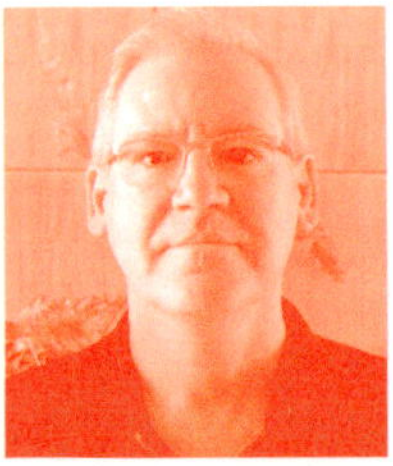

IntechOpen

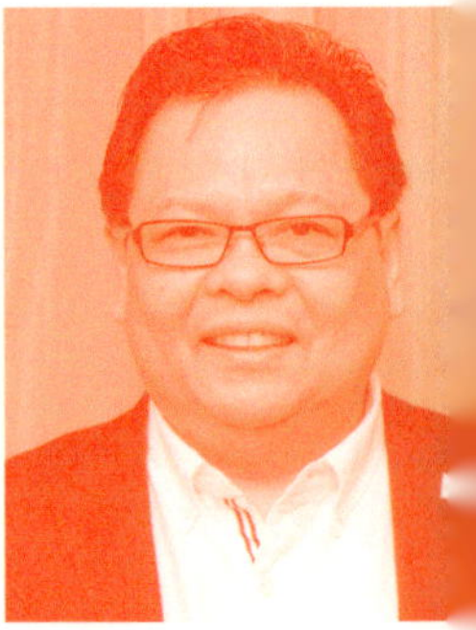
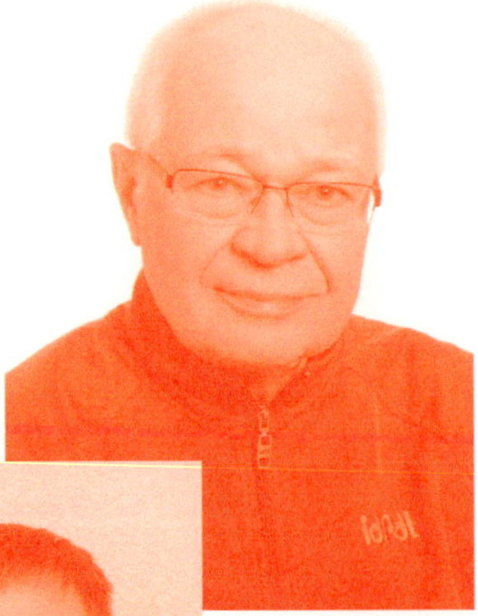
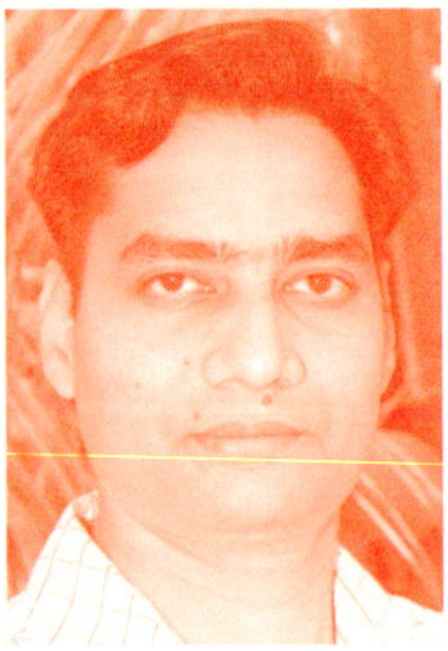
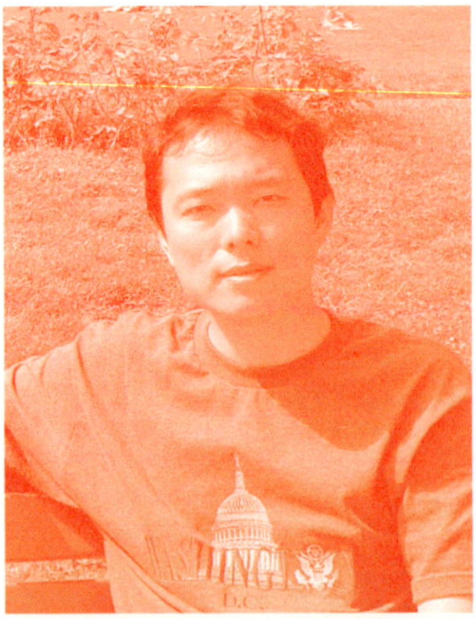
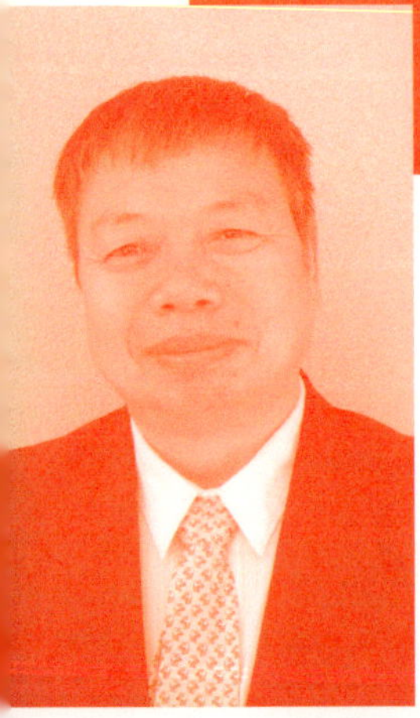
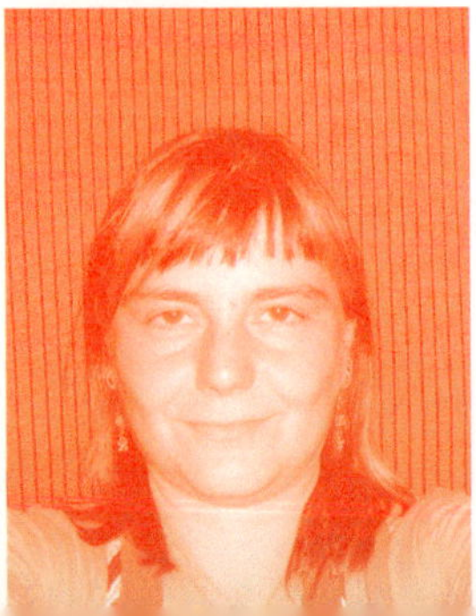

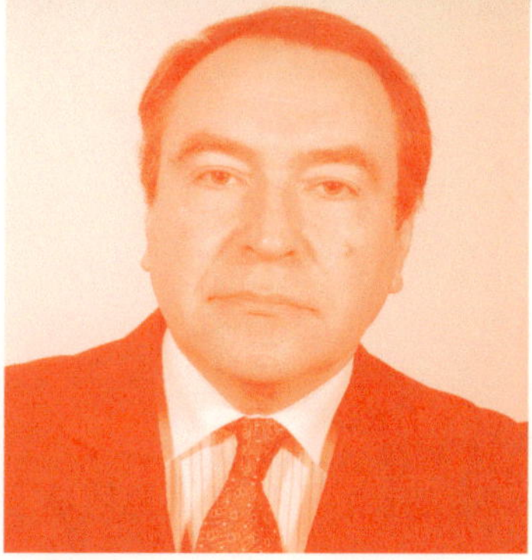

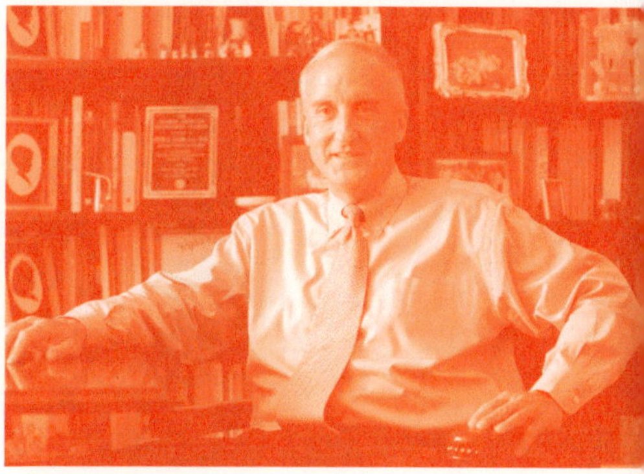

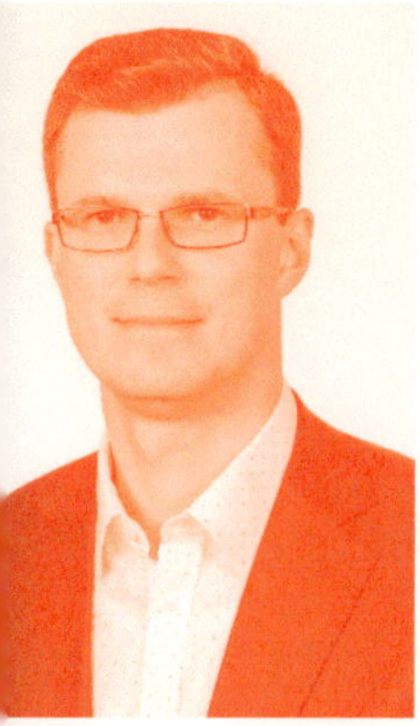

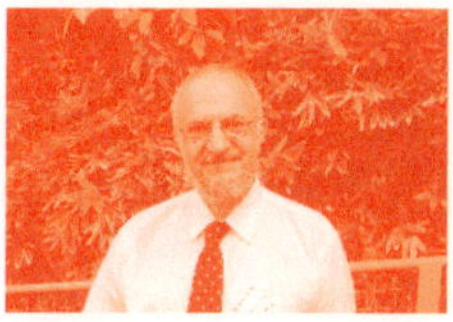

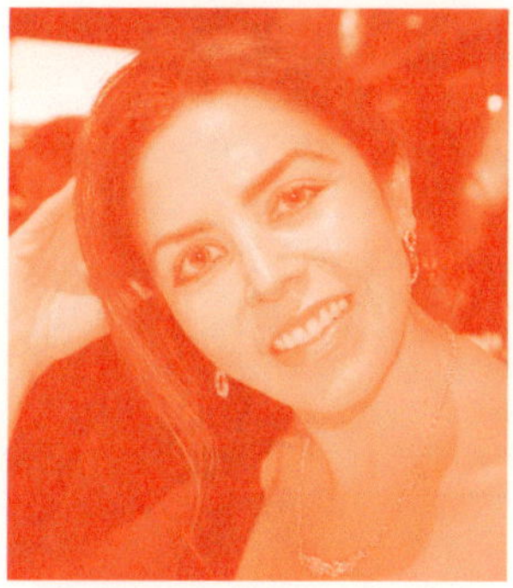

Supporting open minds since 2005

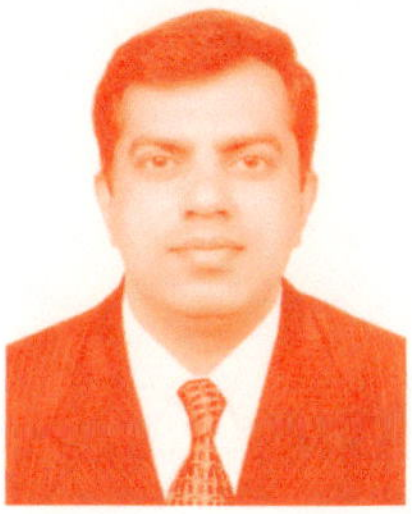

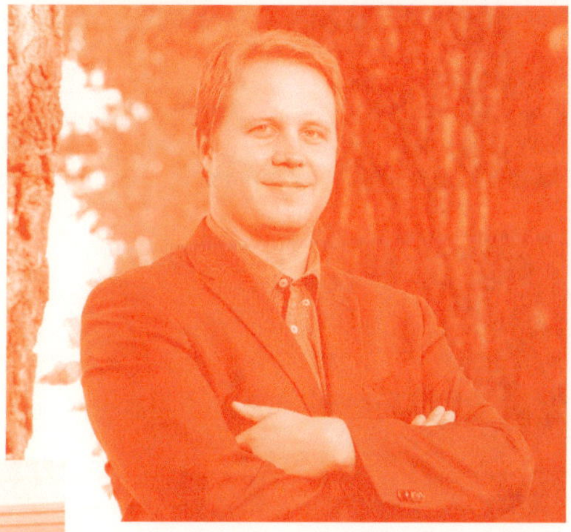

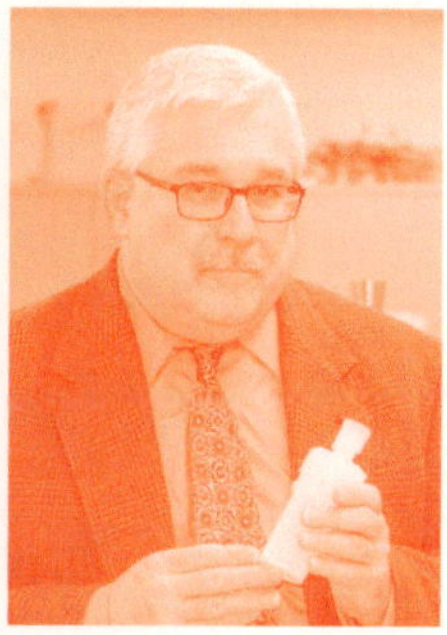

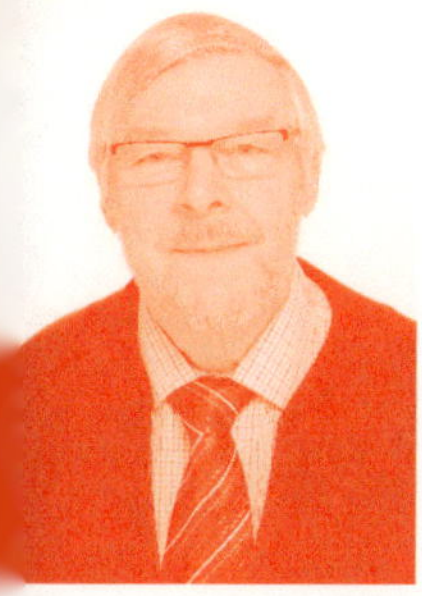

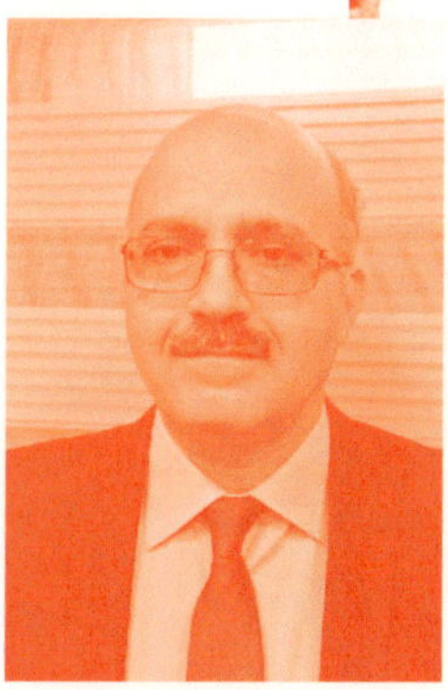

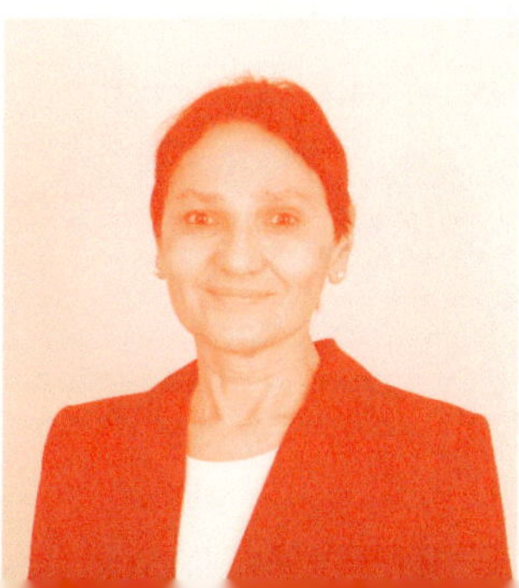

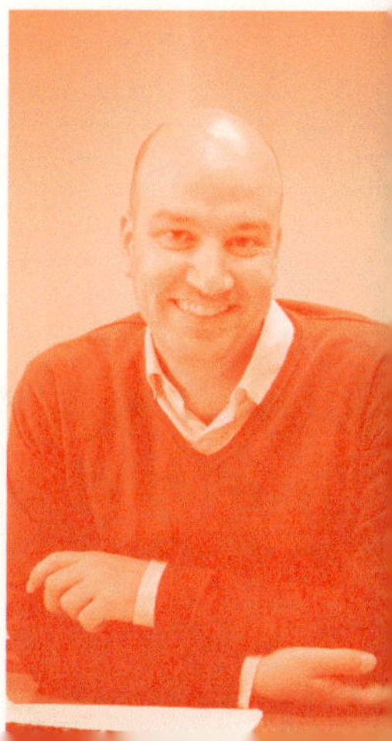

Family Planning and Reproductive Health
http://dx.doi.org/10.5772/intechopen.87291
Edited by Zouhair Amarin and Hassan Abduljabbar

Contributors
Zuzana Judáková, Alhaji A Aliyu, Tukur Dahiru, Javier Cornejo-Reyes, Yaroslava Robles-Bykbaev, Nina Naula, Ana Parra, Blas Garzón, Vladimir Robles-Bykbaev, Jorge Galán, İlkan Kayar, Yakov Y. Yakovlevich Yakovlev, Farok K. Manerov, Olga I. Andriyanova, Olga A. Zagorodnikova, Zouhair Amarin, Mahmoud A. Alfaqih, Sergey A. Dudkin, Nataliya V. Matveeva, Nataliya V. Selivanova, Olga V. Domanskaya

First published in London, United Kingdom, 2020 by IntechOpen
IntechOpen is the global imprint of INTECHOPEN LIMITED, registered in England and Wales, registration number: 11086078, 5 Princes Gate Court, London, SW7 2QJ, United Kingdom
Printed in Croatia

British Library Cataloguing-in-Publication Data
A catalogue record for this book is available from the British Library

Additional hard and PDF copies can be obtained from orders@intechopen.com

Family Planning and Reproductive Health
Edited by Zouhair Amarin and Hassan Abduljabbar
p. cm.
Print ISBN 978-1-83962-538-1
Online ISBN 978-1-83962-539-8
eBook (PDF) ISBN 978-1-83962-540-4

For EU product safety concerns:
IN TECH d.o.o., Prolaz Marije Krucifikse Kozulić 3, 51000 Rijeka, Croatia, info@intechopen.com or visit our website at intechopen.com.

Meet the editors

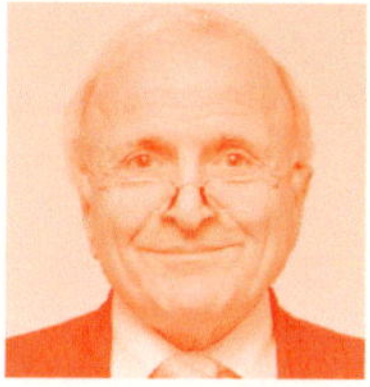

Zouhair Amarin is a Professor of Obstetrics and Gynaecology at the Jordan University of Science and Technology. He was a Lecturer at the University of Glasgow, Senior Lecturer at the University of Nottingham, and Dean of the Faculty of Medicine at Mutah University. Professor Amarin is a Fellow of the Royal College of Obstetricians and Gynaecologists, and the Faculty of Public Health, London. He holds a Master's Degree in Medical Science, Glasgow, and in Medical Education, Maastricht. He is a pioneer in IVF, and was the world's first to develop Microsurgical Epididymis Sperm Aspiration for clinical use. He discovered a surgical procedure for critical Ovarian Hyperstimulation Syndrome. Professor Amarin has published more than 120 papers and has received 8 awards

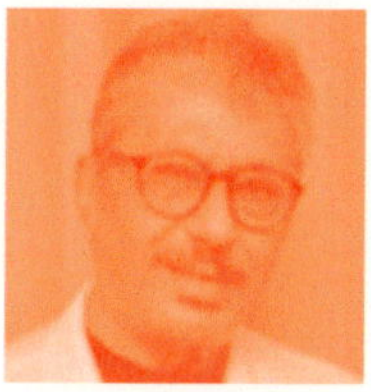

Hassan S Abduljabbar, MD, FRCSC, American Board Diplomat, is a Professor of the Medical College, King Abdulaziz University, and the President of the Saudi Society of Obstetrics and Gynecology. He is the President of the Federation of Arab Gynecology and Obstetrics Societies. His publication list exceeds 50 articles and he is the editor of three books (Steroid Basics (Open Access Books – IntechOpen), Steroid Clinical (Open Access Books – IntechOpen), and Obstetrics (Open Access Books – IntechOpen)). He is also the author of a chapter in a book on the placenta. He is also an author of a 100 MCQ book for medical students. He has four books in the Arabic language.

Contents

Preface

Family planning and taking care of reproductive health allows families to attain their desired number of children and maintain a good family health status. This is achieved by improving the lives of women, children, and families through public health monitoring, scientific assistance, and research.

Many factors need to be considered by couples at certain points in their reproductive period when considering family planning. Choosing a contraceptive method would include the aspects of safety, effectiveness, accessibility, affordability, and acceptability. Family planning reduces the need for abortion and maternal morbidity and mortality.

A woman's reproductive health is delicate and complex. Taking care and making healthy choices can help protect mothers and children. Reproductive health should be high on the priorities list.

The content of this book covers some aspects of family planning and deals with a number of issues that pertain to reproductive health.

The editors are thankful to all the authors for their contributions, and would like to thank Ms. Sara Debeuc, Author Service Manager, and all commissioning editors for their support and advice.

Zouhair O. Amarin
Professor,
Department of Obstetrics and Gynaecology,
Jordan University of Science and Technology,
Irbid, Jordan

Hassan Abduljabbar
King Abdulaziz University,
Saudi Arabia

Section 1

Medical Problems in Obstetrics

Chapter 1

Venous Thromboembolism in the Context of Reproduction: The Royal College of Obstetricians and Gynecologists Recommendations

Zouhair O. Amarin and Mahmoud A. Alfaqih

Abstract

Venous thromboembolism complicates 1–2 of every 1000 deliveries. It may manifest as deep vein thrombosis or pulmonary embolism. Pregnancy-associated venous thromboembolism is an important major cause of maternal morbidity and mortality. Prophylaxis and therapy in pregnancy are complicated by the need to take both fetal and maternal well-being into consideration. Risk factors for venous thromboembolism during pregnancy or the puerperium are multiple. They include, but are not limited to, thrombophilia, multiparity, orthopedic injuries, medical comorbidities, prior venous thromboembolism, smoking, gross varicose veins, age, if older than 35, obesity, multiple pregnancy, preeclampsia, cesarean section, prolonged labor, instrumental vaginal delivery, stillbirth, preterm birth, postpartum hemorrhage, hyperemesis gravidarum, ovarian hyperstimulation syndrome, immobility, long periods of hospitalization, and long haul travel. This chapter is a clinical guide that covers prophylaxis and therapy of pregnancy-associated venous thromboembolism, based on evidence-based research and consensus opinion.

Keywords: obstetrics, pregnancy, prophylaxis, deep vein thrombosis, pulmonary embolism, anticoagulants

1. Introduction

Worldwide, childbearing carries a major risk to the life of women [1]. The Millennium Development Goals (MDGs) were the eight international development goals, and the 192 United Nations states and 23 international organizations had agreed to achieve those goals. Reducing maternal mortality by three quarters over 15 years was a specific part of Goal 5 (Improving Maternal Health) of the eight MDGs [2].

The WHO defines maternal mortality as "the death of a woman while pregnant or within 42 days of termination of pregnancy, irrespective of the duration and site of the pregnancy, from any cause related to or aggravated by the pregnancy or its management but not from accidental or incidental causes" [3].

The maternal mortality ratio (MMR) is a key performance indicator for efforts to improve the safety of mothers before, during, and after childbirth per country. It is the annual number of deaths per 100,000 live births from causes related to or aggravated by pregnancy or its management (not accidental or incidental). It is not to be confused by the maternal mortality rate, which is the number of deaths (direct and indirect) in a given period per 100,000 women of reproductive age during the same time period [1–3].

The regional MMRs for the year 2015 ranged from 11 to 14 for developed regions to 511–652 for sub-Saharan Africa [4].

In a study that estimated the MMR (maternal deaths per 100,000 live births) among Jordanian women aged between 15 and 49 years, there were 76 maternal deaths out of 397,588 live births. The MMR being 19.1. Of these, 43 (56.6%) deaths were caused by hemorrhage, thrombosis, and sepsis [5].

In this same study, avoidable deaths were found in 53.9% of the dead women, 52.6% had substandard care, and 31.5% were poor hospital attenders, having had three or less antenatal visits [5].

Regarding family planning, less than one third of the 76 dead women had ever used any form of contraception [5].

2. Epidemiology

The incidence of venous thromboembolism (VTE) is 1–2 per 1000 pregnancies. In the antenatal period, there is a fivefold higher incidence than nonpregnant women of same age, with deep venous thrombosis (DVT) being more common. In the postnatal period, there is a 20-fold higher incidence, with pulmonary embolism (PE) being more common. Therefore, VTE is considered as one of the leading causes of pregnancy-related deaths [6–10].

3. Pathophysiology

The German physician, anthropologist, pathologist, prehistorian, and "father of modern pathology," Rudolf Virchow (1821–1902), postulated a triad to explain the pathophysiology of the increased incidence of VTE in pregnancy, as follows [11]:

1. Compression of Lt iliac vein by Rt iliac artery or ovarian artery, with 90% DVT on left (vs. 55% nonpregnant), and 70% in iliofemoral veins (vs. 9% nonpregnant)

2. Hypercoagulability

   - Increased clotting factors V, VII, VIII, X, VWf, and fibrinogen

   - Increased resistance to protein C

   - Decreased protein S activity

   - Increased levels of fibrinolytic inhibitors via decreased tissue plasminogen activators and increased plasminogen activator inhibitors

   - Acquired antithrombin III deficiency

3. Endothelial injury

   - Compression by the uterus (and edema)

   - Vascular damage during delivery

There are identifiable risk factors in numerous fatal and nonfatal cases of PE in relation to VTE in pregnancy and puerperium. Therefore, there is a need for risk stratification to determine pharmacological thromboprophylaxis [12].

The risk assessment may be conducted in early pregnancy or prepregnancy at antenatal clinics, at admission to hospital for any reason, intrapartum and immediately postpartum [13].

Hypercoagulability or prothrombotic states increase the risk of thrombosis. Pathologies of this kind are found in a large proportion of women who report one or more episodes of hypercoagulability, such as lower limb or pelvic vein thrombosis, especially when these occur without being provoked by other conditions. A significant number of women have a detectable thrombotic abnormality, where the majority would develop VTE that is related to one or more additional prothrombotic risk factors [13].

4. History

Following the description of the development of thrombosis in 1856 by Virchow, antithrombin deficiency was described in 1965 by Norwegian hematologist Egeberg [14]. Researchers from the Scripps Research Institute described protein C deficiency in 1981 [15]. Researchers at the University of Oklahoma described protein S deficiency in 1984 [16–18].

Graham Hughes, British rheumatologist, described antiphospholipid syndrome 1980s after the finding of antibodies that were associated with SLE and thrombosis [19].

In the 1990s, more studies described genetic thrombophilias and resistance to activated protein C. In 1994, researchers from Leiden, the Netherlands, described a mutation that affected factor V, which made it resistant to activated protein C. Being a genetic defect, it was named factor V Leiden mutation, after its place of discovery [20]. This was followed by the discovery of prothrombin gene mutation by the same group. This mutation results in an increase in prothrombin levels, which may result in some thrombotic episodes [21].

Studies of the human genome and minor gene changes are likely to reveal more genetic abnormalities in cases of hereditary thrombosis [16, 17].

5. Thrombophilia classification

Thrombophilia can be congenital or acquired. Congenital thrombophilia refers to hereditary conditions that increase the tendency to develop thrombosis, while acquired thrombophilia arise later in life [22–24]. The types of thrombophilia are:

Inherited thrombophilias

- Factor V Leiden mutation
- Prothrombin C 20210 mutation (PTM)
- Antithrombin III deficiency
- Protein S deficiency
- Protein C deficiency
- MTHFR mutation (homocysteine)

Acquired thrombophilias - Antiphospholipid syndrome

- Anticardiolipin antibodies
- Lupus anticoagulant antibodies
- Anti β2 glycoprotein 1 antibodies

Thrombophilia is divided into two groups according to risk types:
High risk

- Factor V Leiden mutation, homozygous
- Prothrombin C 20210 mutation, homozygous
- Antithrombin III deficiency
- Antiphospholipid syndrome

Low risk

- Factor V Leiden mutation, heterozygous
- Prothrombin C 20210 mutation, heterozygous
- Protein S deficiency
- Protein C deficiency

Most thrombophilias have no specific therapy, but when thrombosis is recurrent, long-term prophylactic anticoagulation is necessary [22–24].

In general, thrombophilia testing is required for women with history of idiopathic or recurrent episodes of VTE, in addition to women with history of thrombophilia in a first-degree relative [25–28].

6. Risk factors

The risk factors for VTE are:

- Thrombophilia
- Parity of three children or more
- Major orthopedic surgery
- Lower-extremity paralysis due to spinal cord injury
- Fracture of the pelvis, hip, or long bones
- Multiple trauma
- Paraplegia

- Medical comorbidities, for example, cancer, heart failure, SLE, nephrotic syndrome, type I diabetes mellitus with nephropathy, sickle cell disease, and drug addiction
- Prior VTE
- Smoking
- Gross varicose veins
- Age, if older than 35
- Obesity (BMI more than 30)
- Multiple pregnancy
- Preeclampsia
- Cesarean section
- Prolonged labor
- Mid-cavity-assisted vaginal delivery
- Stillbirth
- Preterm birth
- Postpartum hemorrhage
- Hyperemesis and dehydration
- Ovarian hyperstimulation syndrome (OHSS)
- Immobility, such as hospitalization and during long travel
- Oral contraceptives or estrogen treatment for menopause symptoms
- Family history of VTE, especially in a first-degree relative
- Physical inactivity

7. Thromboembolic risk profile

Women who are pregnant or have just had a baby are at greater risk of developing a blood clot. The risk is greater in the presence of other factors. A score is given to each risk factor as follows:

- Previous VTE (except a single event related to major surgery) = 4
- Previous VTE provoked by major surgery = 3
- Known high-risk thrombophilia = 3

- Medical comorbidities = 3
- Obesity BMI ≥ 30 = 1; BMI ≥ 40 = 2
- Cesarean section in labor = 2
- Any surgical procedure in pregnancy or puerperium except immediate repair of the perineum + = 3
- Hyperemesis =3
- OHSS (first trimester only) = 4
- Any other = 1

8. Thromboprophylaxis

Prophylaxis is administered according to the risk assessment's total score as follows:

- ≥4 antenatal: prophylaxis from first trimester and puerperium
- 3 antenatal: prophylaxis from 28 weeks and puerperium
- ≥2 postnatal: prophylaxis for at least 10 days

There should be a lower postnatal threshold for prophylaxis than antenatally as risk per day is higher and duration of risk is shorter.

Women with antithrombin deficiency are often on long term oral anticoagulants, and extra advice is necessary as follows:

- Prophylaxis with a higher dose of low molecular weight heparin (LMWH) antenatally and 6 weeks postpartum or until return to oral therapy
- Anti-Xa monitoring (4-h peak levels 0.5–1.0 iu/ml)
- Possible antithrombin therapy at start of labor or prior to cesarean section (CS)

Women with previous recurrent VTE need extra advice as follows:

- Higher doses of LMWH
- If on long-term warfarin or other oral anticoagulants
    - Counsel about the risks to the fetus
    - Stop oral therapy, change to LMWH, within 2 weeks of the missed period and before the sixth week of pregnancy
- Not on oral anticoagulants: LMWH as soon as pregnancy test is +ve

There are other first trimester risk factors for VTE that include:

- Women with hyperemesis should be considered for prophylaxis with LMWH. Discontinue when it resolves
- Women with OHSS need prophylaxis with LMWH in the first trimester
- In vitro fertilization pregnancy and three other risk factors need prophylaxis, with LMWH starting in the first trimester

Thromboprophylaxis should be interrupted for delivery in the case of any vaginal bleeding or labor, no further LMWH is administered [13].

When regional anesthetic techniques are considered, the following should be implemented:

- Avoid for 12 h after the previous prophylactic dose of LMWH
- No LMWH for 4 h after spinal or after epidural catheter removal
- No catheter removal for 12 h of injection
- If on a therapeutic LMWH, it should be avoided for 24 h after the last dose

With regard to prophylaxis in labor and delivery:

- Women on antenatal LMWH having an elective CS should receive prophylactic LMWH on the day prior to CS
- The morning dose on CS day should be omitted, the operation should take place that morning
- The first prophylactic dose of LMWH should be given 4–6 h after vaginal delivery, 6–12 h after CS (if no postpartum hemorrhage or regional anesthesia)
- Women with previous VTE and postpartum thromboprophylaxis should receive LMWH or warfarin for at least 6 weeks regardless of mode of delivery
- Women that undergo emergency CS should receive cover with LMWH for 10 days. The same applies for elective CS in the presence of additional risk factors

With regard to LMWH:

- It is the agent of choice for antenatal and postnatal prophylaxis
- For prophylaxis, the doses based on booking or most recent weight
- Platelet count needs monitoring only if prior exposure to unfractionated heparin (UFH)
- No need for monitoring of anti-Xa levels if LMWH is for prophylaxis

- LMWH should be reduced in renal impairment
- LMWH is safe in breastfeeding

Unfractionated heparin should be considered in cases of very high risk of thrombosis, and an increased risk of hemorrhage, UFH may be used peripartum, especially if regional anesthetic may be required. If UFH is used, platelet count should be monitored every 2–3 days from days 4–14 or until UFH is stopped [13].

The molecular weight (MW) of natural heparin is 5000–40,000 Daltons. The MWH is less than 8000 Daltons. The half-life of UFH is 1–2 h, whereas LMWH is 4–8 h.

Danaparoid and fondaparinux are used only when heparins cannot be used due to heparin induced thrombocytopenia or a skin allergy and perhaps should be prescribed by a hematologist with expertise in hemostasis in pregnancy. Regional anesthesia is to be avoided because of 24-h half-life [13].

Low-dose aspirin is not recommended for thromboprophylaxis in obstetric patients [13].

Dextran should be avoided antenatally and intrapartum because it is less effective than LMWH, increases the risk of bleeding and anaphylaxis that has been associated with uterine hypertonus, fetal distress, fetal neurological abnormalities, and fetal death [13].

Oral thrombin and Xa inhibitors are non-vitamin K antagonist oral anticoagulants (NOACs) that should be avoided in pregnant women and are not currently recommended in breastfeeding [13].

Warfarin crosses placenta. If used between 6 and 12 weeks, there is a dose-dependent risk of embryopathy, as 5% of fetuses develop nasal bridge hypoplasia, heart defects, vetriculomegaly, agenesis of corpus callosum, and stippled epiphysis. In addition, it is associated with an increased incidence of spontaneous miscarriage, stillbirth, neurological problems, and fetal and maternal hemorrhage. Its use in pregnancy is restricted to women with mechanical heart valves. It is safe in breastfeeding, and may convert from LMWH to warfarin postpartum when risk of hemorrhage is low, 5–7 days after delivery [13].

The suggested daily thromboprophylactic doses for antenatal and postnatal LMWH are weight dependent. For the average weight of 50–90 kg, the doses of enoxaparin, dalteparin and tinzaparin are 20 mg, 2500 and 3500 iu, respectively.

Contraindications to LMWH are the following:

- Known bleeding disorder
- Previous or current allergic reactions
- Active antenatal or postpartum bleeding
- High risk of major hemorrhage
- Thrombocytopenia $<75 \times 10^9/l$
- Acute stroke in previous 4 weeks
- Severe renal or liver disease
- Uncontrolled hypertension

9. Acute management of VTE

Diagnosis of acute VTE requires high index of suspicion. Its symptoms and signs are:

- Leg pain and swelling, usually unilateral
- Lower abdominal pain
- PE: dyspnea, chest pain, hemoptysis and collapse
- Low-grade pyrexia and leukocytosis can occur

The symptoms or signs of VTE require objective testing and treatment with LMWH expeditiously. If DVT remains untreated, 20% will develop pulmonary embolism (PE), which, in pregnancy is fatal in 15%, and in 66% of these, death will result within 30 min of the embolic event [13], that is, there are three deaths per 100 DVTs.

The investigations for suspected DVT include compression duplex ultrasound, CBC, coagulation screen, kidney, and liver function tests. D-dimer and thrombophilia screen are not recommended prior to therapy [13].

The following is recommended in the initial anticoagulant treatment of VTE in pregnancy:

- Clinically suspected DVT or PE, LMWH immediately until the diagnosis is excluded by objective testing, unless strongly contraindicated
- LMWHs are not associated with an increased risk of severe PPH
- Lower risk of heparin-induced osteoporosis with LMWH versus UFHs
- LMWH titrated against booking or early pregnancy weight. Insufficient evidence for once daily or in two divided doses
- No routine peak anti-Xa activity of LMWH except in weight < 50 kg and > 90 kg or with renal impairment or recurrent VTE
- Routine platelet count monitoring should not be carried out
- Initial management of DVT, leg elevation, and a graduated elastic compression stocking. Mobilization with graduated elastic compression stockings
- Temporary IVC filter peripartum for patients with iliac vein VTE to reduce the risk of PE or recurrent PE despite adequate anticoagulation
- Therapeutic doses of subcutaneous LMWH for the remainder of pregnancy and for at least 6 weeks postnatally and for at least 3 months of treatment in total
- Because of their adverse effects on the fetus, warfarin should not be used for antenatal VTE treatment

With regard to anticoagulation during labor and delivery, the following should apply:

- VTE at term: consider IV UFH, more easily manipulated
- If on LMWH for maintenance and in early labor, no further heparin
- Planned elective CS or induction of labor, discontinue LMWH maintenance 24 h in advance
- No regional anesthesia or analgesia for 24 h after therapeutic LMWH dose
- No LMWH for 4 h after spinal anesthesia or after epidural catheter removal. No epidural catheter removal within 12 h of the most recent injection

The initial daily therapeutic doses of enoxaparin, dalteparin, and tinzaparin are weight dependent, their initial doses for the average women between 50 and 90 kg are 60 mg twice daily or 90 mg once daily, 6000 iu twice daily or 1200 iu once daily, 175 iu/kg once daily, respectively [13].

For anticoagulated patients undergoing CS, the following is recommended:

- If therapeutic doses of LMWH: wound drains (abdominal and rectus sheath) at CS. Skin closure with interrupted sutures for drainage of any hematoma
- Women at high risk of hemorrhage, in whom continued heparin is considered essential, manage with IV UFH until the risk factors for hemorrhage resolve

The regimen for the IV UFH is:

- Loading dose of 80 u/kg, followed by a continuous IV infusion of 18 u/kg/h
- In case of thrombolysis, omit loading dose and infusion starts at 18 u/kg/h
- Mandatory APTT 4–6 h after loading dose, 6 h after dose change, then daily when in therapeutic range. The target is 1.5–2.5 X control value
- The infusion rate should be adjusted according to the APTT

To monitor heparin therapy in pregnancy, routine measurement of peak anti-Xa activity of LMWH for acute VTE, if body weight is less than 50 and more than 90 kg, in renal impairment or recurrent VTE is required. Postoperative women receiving UFH should have platelet count every 2–3 days until heparin is stopped. Women are taught to self-inject LMWH and to safely dispose needles etc. [13].

In cases of acute PE, CXR, compression duplex ultrasound and ECG should be performed. ECG may show "S1Q3T3" pattern (large S wave in lead I, Q wave in lead III, and inverted T wave in lead III), Rt BBB, M wave V1 and broad S V6, due to acute right heart strain [13].

If DVT is present, no further investigations are required, and treatment should continue [13].

In suspected PE without symptoms and signs of DVT, CT pulmonary angiogram or V/Q lung scan should be performed. If CXR is abnormal with suspicion of PE, CTPA is better than V/Q scan. In cases of normal ventilation with multiple segmental perfusion deficits, the probability of PE is 80%. There is a slightly increased risk of childhood Ca but lower risk of maternal breast Ca than CTPA. The absolute risk is very small in both [13].

Anticoagulation should be continued until PE is definitively excluded [13].

In acute PE, it is recommended that:

- Shocked women who are pregnant or in the puerperium are managed individually regarding IV UFH, thrombolytic therapy or thoracotomy and embolectomy
- Multidisciplinary involvement of senior physicians, obstetricians, surgeons, and radiologists
- IV UFH is preferred in massive PE with cardiovascular compromise
- Urgent portable ECG or CTPA within 1 h of presentation. Immediate thrombolysis should be considered
- Maternal resuscitation as per immediate life support. Cardiopulmonary resuscitation in a left lateral tilt. Perimortem CS by 5 min if resuscitation is unsuccessful and the pregnancy is more than 20 weeks

10. Key points

- LMWH is the agent of choice for antenatal prophylaxis
- Score ≥ 4 antenatal: prophylaxis in first trimester and 6 weeks postnatally
- Score = 3 antenatal: prophylaxis from 28 weeks and 6 weeks postnatally
- Score ≥ 2 postnatal: prophylaxis for a minimum of 10 days
- Women on antenatal prophylaxis are for postnatal prophylaxis for 6 weeks
- Women with symptoms or signs of VTE should have LMWH until the diagnosis is excluded by objective testing, unless strongly contraindicated
- All women should undergo a documented thromboembolic risk profile for VTE before conception and in early pregnancy
- The documented thromboembolic risk profile should be repeated if admission to hospital is required or if an intercurrent medical condition does occur
- A repetition of the thromboembolic risk profile is required intrapartum and in the immediate postpartum period

Author details

Zouhair O. Amarin[1]* and Mahmoud A. Alfaqih[2]

1 Department of Obstetrics and Gynaecology, Faculty of Medicine, Jordan University of Science and Technology, Irbid, Jordan

2 Department of Physiology and Biochemistry, Faculty of Medicine, Jordan University of Science and Technology, Irbid, Jordan

*Address all correspondence to: zoamarin@hotmail.com

References

[1] Ozimek J, Kilpatrick S. Maternal mortality in the twenty-first century. Obstetrics and Gynecology Clinics of North America. 2018;**45**(2):175-186. DOI: 10.1016/j.ogc.2018.01.004

[2] Campbel A. Update on the United Nations millennium development goals. Journal of Obstetric, Gynecologic, and Neonatal Nursing. 2017;**46**(3):e48-e55. DOI: 10.1016/j.jogn.2016.11.010

[3] Say L, Chou D, Gemmill AM, et al. Global causes of maternal death: A WHO systematic analysis. The Lancet Global Health. 2014;**2**(6):e323-e333. DOI: 10.1016/S2214-109X (14)70227-X

[4] Alkema L, Chou D, Hogan D, et al. Global, regional, and national levels and trends in maternal mortality between 1990 and 2015, with scenario-based projections to 2030: A systematic analysis by the UN maternal mortality estimation inter-agency group. Lancet. 2016;**387**(10017):462-474. DOI: 10.1016/S0140-6736(15)00838-7

[5] Amarin Z, Khader Y, Okour A, Jaddou H, Al-Qutob R. National maternal mortality ratio for Jordan, 2007-2008. International Journal of Gynaecology and Obstetrics. 2010;**111**:152-156

[6] Knight M. UKOSS. Antenatal pulmonary embolism: Risk factors, management and outcomes. BJOG. 2008;**115**:453-461

[7] Heit J, Kobbervig C, James A, et al. Trends in the incidence of venous thromboembolism during pregnancy or postpartum: A 30-year population-based study. Annals of Internal Medicine. 2005;**143**:697-706

[8] Sultan A, West J, Tata L, et al. Risk of first venous thromboembolism in and around pregnancy: A population-based cohort study. British Journal of Haematology. 2012;**156**:366-373

[9] Pomp E, Lenselink A, Rosendaal F, et al. Pregnancy, the postpartum period and prothrombotic defects: Risk of venous thrombosis in the MEGA study. Journal of Thrombosis and Haemostasis. 2008;**6**:632-637

[10] Jackson E, Curtis M. Risk of venous thromboembolism during the postpartum period: A systematic review. Obstetrics and Gynecology. 2011;**117**:691-703

[11] Kumar D, Hanlin E, Glurich I, et al. Virchow's contribution to the understanding of thrombosis and cellular biology. Clinical Medicine & Research. 2010

[12] Doherty S. Pulmonary embolism an update. Australian Family Physician. 2017 Nov;**46**(11):816-820

[13] Royal College of Obstetricians and Gynaecologists. Thromboembolic Disease in Pregnancy and the Puerperium: Acute Management. Green-Top Guideline No. 37a. London: RCOG; 2015

[14] Egeberg O. Inherited antithrombin deficiency causing thrombophilia. Thrombosis et Diathesis Haemorrhagica. 1965;**13**(2):516-530. DOI: 10.1055/s-0038-1656297

[15] Griffin JH, Evatt B, Zimmerman TS, Kleiss AJ, Wideman C. Deficiency of protein C in congenital thrombotic disease. The Journal of Clinical Investigation. 1981;**68**(5):1370-1373. DOI: 10.1172/JCI110385. PMC 370934. PMID 6895379

[16] Dahlbäck B. Advances in understanding pathogenic mechanisms of thrombophilic disorders. Blood. 2008;**112**(1):19-27. DOI: 10.1182/blood-2008-01-077909

[17] Rosendaal FR, Reitsma PH. Genetics of venous thrombosis. Journal

of Thrombosis and Haemostasis. 2009;**7**(Suppl 1):301-304. DOI: 10.1111/j.1538-7836.2009.03394.x

[18] Comp PC, Esmon CT. Recurrent venous thromboembolism in patients with a partial deficiency of protein S. The New England Journal of Medicine. 1984;**311**(24):1525-1528. DOI: 10.1056/NEJM198412133112401. PMID 6239102

[19] Sanna G, D'Cruz D, Cuadrado MJ. Cerebral manifestations in the 6antiphospholipid (Hughes) syndrome. Rheumatic Diseases Clinics of North America. 2006;**32**(3):465-490. DOI: 10.1016/j.rdc.2006.05.010. PMID 16880079

[20] Bertina RM, Koeleman BP, Koster T, et al. Mutation in blood coagulation factor V associated with resistance to activated protein C. Nature. 1994;**369**(6475):64-67

[21] Poort SR, Rosendaal FR, Reitsma PH, Bertina RM. A common genetic variation in the 3′-untranslated region of the prothrombin gene is associated with elevated plasma prothrombin levels and an increase in venous thrombosis. Blood. 1996;**88**(10):3698-3703. DOI: 10.1182/blood.V88.10.3698.bloodjournal88103698

[22] Čingerová L, Kučeráková M, Vnitr L. Thrombophilia. Winter. 2016;**62**(12):985-989

[23] Middeldorp S. Inherited thrombophilia: A double-edged sword. Hematology. American Society of Hematology. Education Program. 2016;**2016**(1):1-9. DOI: 10.1182/asheducation-2016.1.1

[24] Connors J. Thrombophilia testing and venous thrombosis. The New England Journal of Medicine. 2017;**377**(12):1177-1187. DOI: 10.1056/NEJMra1700365

[25] Simcox L, Ormesher L, Tower C, et al. Thrombophilia and pregnancy complications. International Journal of Molecular Sciences. 2015;**16**(12):28418-28428. DOI: 10.3390/ijms161226104

[26] Moll S. Clinical-practical aspects. Journal of Thrombosis and Thrombolysis. 2015;**39**(3):367-378. DOI: 10.1007/s11239-015-1197-3

[27] Stern R, Al-Samkari H, Connors J. Thrombophilia evaluation in pulmonary embolism. Current Opinion in Cardiology. 2019 Nov;**34**(6):603-609. DOI: 10.1097/HCO.0000000000000668

[28] Stevens S, Woller S, Bauer K, et al. Guidance for the evaluation and treatment of hereditary and acquired thrombophilia. Journal of Thrombosis and Thrombolysis. 2016;**41**(1):154-164. DOI: 10.1007/s11239-015-1316-1

Section 2

Family Planning in the Era of Information Technology

Chapter 2

The Role of Information Technologies in Natural Family Planning

Zuzana Judáková

Abstract

Freedom is needed in family planning and in the decision on how many children the couple will have, not to be influenced by a third person, political situations, or religious conviction. There is a need for information, education, and communication about possibilities in natural family planning, in order to be able to choose the right way, because there are many options even without side effects. Nowadays, we can add to these traditional possibilities of natural family planning also information technologies and electronic devices, which are increasingly available to a large portion of the population. Their reliability, with correct usage, is comparable to the barrier methods and in some cases to hormonal contraceptive methods. Next development of these devices can more increase their reliability. Of course, the active approach of users is needed.

Keywords: natural family planning, basal body temperature, cervical mucus, symptothermal method, information technologies, electronic devices, digitized records, application, evaluation, reliability, price

1. Introduction

"Natural family planning (NFP) is a term used to describe methods of planning or preventing pregnancy based on observation of naturally occurring signs and symptoms of the fertile and infertile phases of the menstrual cycle. People who use NFP to avoid or delay pregnancy abstain from intercourse on potentially fertile days. Those wanting to achieve pregnancy use NFP to identify the fertile phase and hence maximize the probability of pregnancy. Techniques include the basal body temperature method, the cervical mucus (Billings') method, the symptothermal method, and the calendar or rhythm method (Ogino-Knaus). It is important to note that NFP is not a method of contraception but rather a technique for determining the fertile period; abstinence during this period is what prevents pregnancy. The methods are thus likely to be of interest to people who, for any reason, do not wish to use mechanical or pharmacological contraceptives" [1]. This is the definition given by the World Health Organization in their publication about NFP. To this definition, some additional notes have to be added: NFP is a manifestation of a responsible attitude towards family and own health, and it helps a woman to know how her body works, which has many benefits not only in family planning. The human body is the complex sensitive system. If the woman knows her own body and makes regular self-monitoring, she knows when everything is alright and when it is needed to seek expert help. We must not forget either the psychological side of NFP, because the intercourse is not only a physiological act but it influences an individual's psychological state or soul and a mutual relationship, especially in marriage. If both partners identify the use of NFP methods, this strengthens their mutual bond. The use of these methods is becoming a lifestyle. No known side effects and no external factors that affect or damage this sophisticated, naturally designed fertility mechanism are also a benefit. The disadvantages include more demanding, but not impossible, use during nonstandard situations such as breastfeeding, menopause, the medications affecting the menstrual cycle, previous contraception use, and irregular cycles. The solution of some disadvantages and increase in the comfort of using NFP methods bring information technologies in the form of electronic devices and applications.

2. Natural family planning methods

Natural family planning methods are those that don't use a chemical or mechanical contraceptive. The basis of their use is the observation of fertility symptoms and determination of fertile and infertile windows and periodical abstinence practice. Each method uses another symptom singly or a combination of symptoms.

2.1 Cervical mucus method

This method is known as the Billings Ovulation Method (BOM). The method is based on the observation of the structure and density of cervical mucus. Cervical mucus is a normal, healthy secretion of the cervix formed by the effects of estrogen hormones, usually appears on the genitals a few days before ovulation and at the time of ovulation, and is usually lost after ovulation. The cervical mucus is a very positive sign of fertility as it provides the sperm with nutrition and a suitable environment for movement. Observations are indicated in **Figure 1** to obtain an accurate record of the course of the cycle and the onset of fertile days. The method has four rules: three preovulatory rules and one after ovulation rule—the rule of the peak. Method requirements are an accurate observation, accurate records, and motivation and cooperation of the couple. By following the rules of the method to delayed conception, efficiency is greater than 99% [1]. Another modification of this cervical mucus method is Creighton Model FertilityCare System (CrMS); however, it uses a different picture dictionary (PD) and standardized terminology. CrMS forms the basis for Natural Procreative Technology (NaProTECHNOLOGY) successfully used for achieving pregnancy in infertility problems and miscarriage. In addition, NaProTECHNOLOGY uses a series of sonographic examinations during different parts of the cycle and repeated blood tests to identify the causes of infertility. The main idea of this type of infertility treatment is a minimal intervention in the female cycle and the effort to avoid hormonal stimulation or in vitro fertilization (IVF), in accordance with NFP [2].

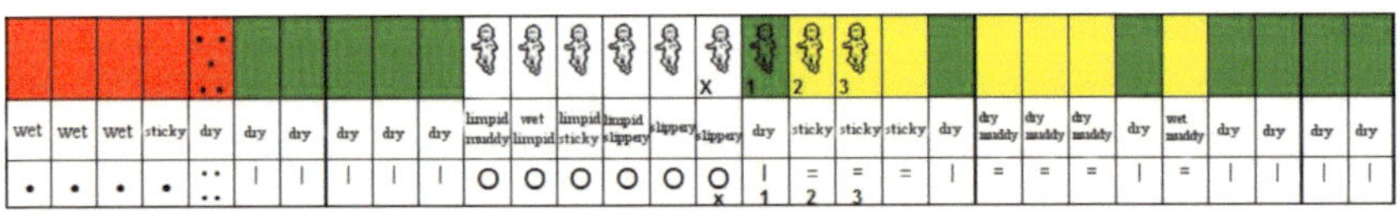

Figure 1.
BOM record table.

2.2 Basal temperature method

Basal body temperature (BBT) is the temperature of a relaxed human body measured in a moment after waking up after a minimum of 6 h of night sleep, unaffected by food, drink, or physical exertion. After ovulation, the ruptured follicle becomes a yellow corpus luteum and begins to produce the hormone progesterone, which causes a postovulatory increase in BBT. This ascension lasts until the next menstruation. Two-level temperature curves are therefore typical for a healthy fertile woman, as shown in **Figure 2**. There are precise rules to record the temperature curve; temperature is measured to a minimum of two decimal places. The BBT shift typically occurs 1 day after the day of ovulation, so the fertile phase can be determined 5 days before the temperature shift and 2 days after it. This calculation of fertile window includes twofold ovulation and sperm life span. Approximately 1 day before ovulation, a decrease of BBT can be observed typically [3].

2.3 Symptothermal method

The combination of both previous methods, cervical mucus and basal temperature method, is the symptothermal method that was developed by Austrian Dr. Josef Rötzer [4]. As the name itself suggests, the method used to menstrual cycle evaluation basal body temperature and symptoms of fertility, viz., cervical mucus and cervix changes. Another symptom can be used too, e.g., breast tenderness and lower abdominal pain. All observed fertile symptoms are recorded in special record table and evaluated by 11 rules—4 rules for specifying infertility before ovulation and 7 rules for specifying postovulatory infertility. For evaluating one cycle, it is not needed to use every rule. The most appropriate rule applies. The reliability of the method was determined by the Pearl Index, PI 0.4 [5, 6].

2.4 Calendar/rhythm method

The calendar method (sometimes called the Ogino-Knaus method) assumes that a woman will have a regular menstrual cycle. The observed symptom is only the first day of menstruation. From the length of the previous cycles (shortest and longest), it determines the beginning and end of the fertile period of the following cycle according to certain rules (each author states slightly different rules). This method is obsolete and unreliable mainly for irregular cycles. Pearl Index of this method was estimated on 18.5 + 1.8 [7].

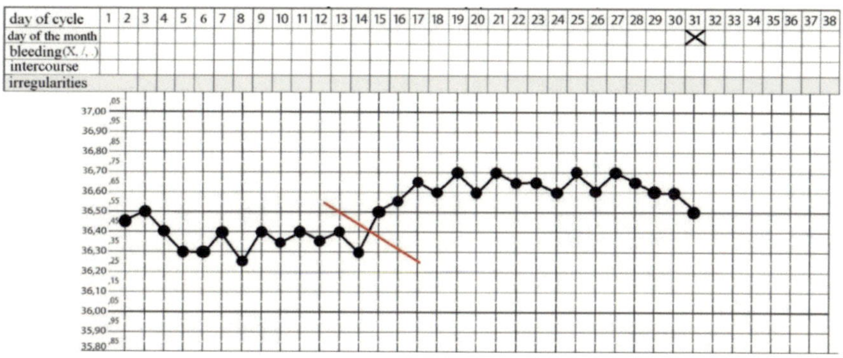

Figure 2.
BBT records.

The successful use of NFP methods clearly involves a thorough study of the rules of a particular method and their consistent adherence. The success rate decreases significantly with careless use and application of the rules. Human factor failure is the most common cause of an unplanned pregnancy. Therefore, there are many books, courses, and professional teacher pairs, with a certificate for each method, that teach the rules of using NFP methods and usually offer free evaluation support of fertility symptoms. The practical experience of teacher couples using a particular method is very helpful.

3. Information technologies and electronic devices

New technologies are also entering NFP. There is a hope that it will make it possible to reduce the length of the required abstinence to the necessary time. These include, in the first place, devices for measuring hormone levels in the urine (e.g., Persona, ClearBlue Easy Fertility Monitor). The preliminary results of their testing in practice are encouraging, but their effectiveness has not yet exceeded the level achieved by the symptothermal method. There are also minicomputers that measure and evaluate the basal body temperature (e.g., Lady-Comp, Daysy, iFertracker, OvuSense) or the temperature and luteinizing hormone content in the urine and cervical mucus (Cyclotest myWay). Their advantage is that the woman does not have to keep records because they are stored in the computer memory but otherwise in principle do not differ from the temperature method. Miniature microscopes for monitoring saliva crystallization (e.g., Lady Q) have proven unreliable and can only be recommended to couples who wish to conceive.

3.1 Cyclotest myWay

For evaluating fertile days by Cyclotest (**Figure 3**) the basis is the measurement of the basal body temperature. For increasing the safety of this device, the two fertile symptoms can be included—ovulation test or quality of cervical mucus. The cycle computers follow exactly the symptothermal methodology. Even an irregular cycle that is still within the normal range can be reliably evaluated, and it is possible to record the cycle length from 23 to 45 days. When irregularities occur, the temperature should not be measured. Alternatively, continue measuring and manually note the results for that particular day as a disruption. After pregnancy the device can be used as soon as the menstruation is regular again and woman is not nursing at night.

The cycles can be saved as a PDF file via Cyclotest mySoftware, the software comes for free. The computer alerts of possible ovarian insufficiency in the last

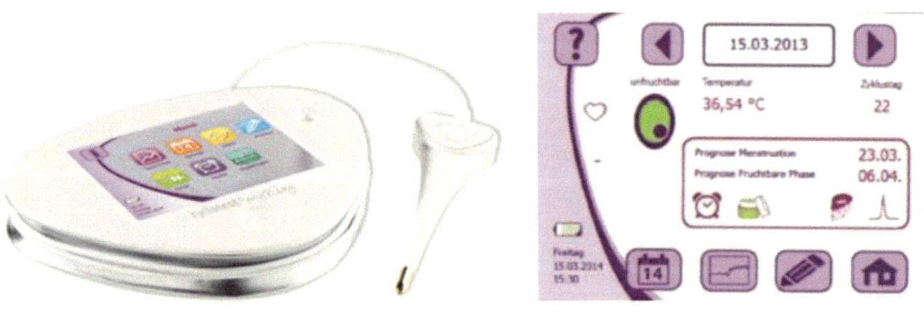

Figure 3.
Cyclotest myWay device and information on screen [8].

12 cycles are stored and offer additional function skincare, which shows what type of cream is most applicable for which days of the cycle. The settings can be switched between the two modes—child planning and cycle control. One computer can be used for two objectives. In the child planning mode, the following additional functions will be activated:

- Indication of possible luteal phase deficiency
- Pregnancy display
- Birth planner
- Display of the highly fertile days

Apart from that, the menu only differs in coloration. In the "child planning" mode, the dominant color is magenta, and in the "cycle control" mode, it is violet. The price of these devices on the manufacturer's website is $ 333, and replacement of measuring probe costs $ 56. In terms of reliability, manufacturers refers to the reliability of the symptothermal method; they do not specify reliability in percentage or Pearl Index for this device especially [8].

3.2 Lady-Comp

Lady-Comp is an intelligent fertility tracker/minicomputer designed to determine fertile and infertile days by morning BBT in the mouth 60 s every morning. The Lady-Comp works on the basis of more than 1 million cycles with statistical data to determine fertile and infertile days, with an accuracy of 99.3% [9], and the day of ovulation. Lady-Comp observes the individual cycle and determines fertility for the next 24 h. It correctly evaluates complicated and irregular cycles and identifies and eliminates unlikely temperature measurements, e.g., fever. The device displays temperature, menstruation, fertility: red, fertile day; green, infertile day; and yellow, learning phase or uncertainty. It offers the possibility to write personal data into the calendar, download and print raw data or upload it into the website, and get a full analysis of cycle, all averages, and a lot of interesting charts and graphs. Lady-Comp can be upgraded to Lady-Comp Baby, which works with over 5 million cycle data and has extra features to plan a baby naturally:

- CLI (low corpus luteum function)
- Forecast hits for 20 cycles
- Documentation of intercourse
- Indication of possible pregnancy after 4–5 days
- Indication of probable pregnancy after 15 days
- Conception date and birth date

Pearly is a simpler and less expensive solution from the same manufacturer. Pearly is a pocket-size fertility tracker working on the same way as Lady-Comp; however, it has fewer functions. Fertility status is evaluated via color lights, as

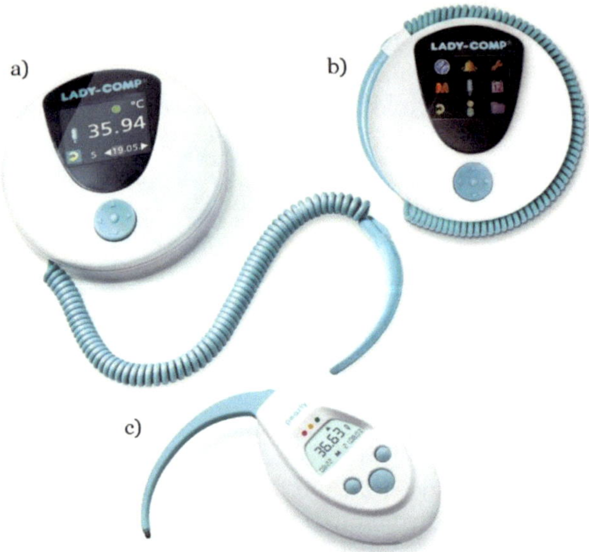

Figure 4.
(a) Lady-Comp, (b) Lady-Comp baby, and (c) Pearly [10].

well as in Lady-Comp (**Figure 4**). The price of these devices ranges from $ 375 for Pearly, $ 455 for Lady-Comp to $ 545 for Lady-Comp Baby. Replacement of measuring probe costs $ 56 [11].

3.3 Daysy

Daysy uses the same evaluating algorithm as Lady-Comp and has the same reliability of 99.3%. Thermometer with accuracy 0.01°C records the BBT every morning in 60 s. The device itself does not have a display; it has only one activation button and three control lights. Information about fertility are separate—past data are only in the phone app, and actual fertility status is displayed in the device as color light. Daysy (**Figure 5**) is CE certified and is a Class I medical device. It has exceptional design and appearance, but for more detailed information, it is necessary to use the mobile application. The manufacturer's price is $ 333, and the application is for free [12].

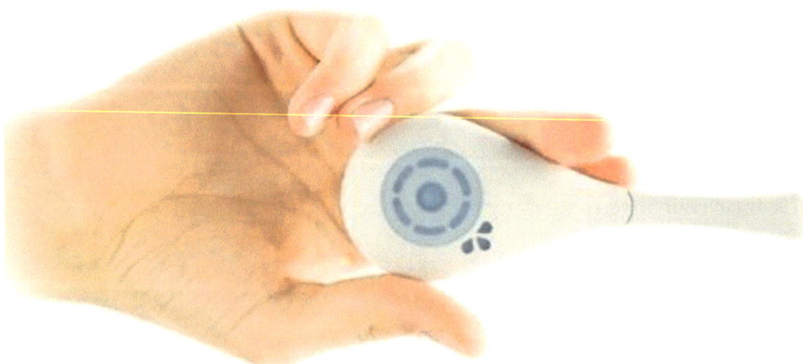

Figure 5.
Daysy device [13].

3.4 iFertracker

The iFertracker is applicable for both the fertility awareness method (FAM) and the symptothermal method of natural family planning. The device itself is actually a thermometer that captures core temperature opposed to the skin or environmental temperature which is stuck to the armpit by means of double-sided medical tape. iFertracker monitors temperature continuously overnight and collects 20,000 data points with an accuracy of 0.01°C in a single night. The device identifies invalid data, such as getting up in the middle of the night, and works around different sleeping schedules to provide flexibility without disturbing the integrity of data. It is necessary to send data from the thermometer to the mobile app every morning via Bluetooth. The application automatically charts data and provides a daily fertility snapshot. The application also offers notifications for when the pair should try to conceive and allows exporting the BBT chart from directly within the app. The manufacturer recommends keeping track of factors like sexual activity, stress, cervical mucus quality, and sleep to increase the accuracy of ovulation prediction. Change in these habits can cause natural BBT fluctuation and impact the menstrual cycle. The cost of iFertracker and 90 double-sided adhesive patches is $ 129.00, 60 pieces of replacement disposable medical patches cost $ 14.99, and the application is for free. The manufacturer does not report reliability or any scientific studies on their product [14].

On the market other thermometers are also available which measure continuous core body temperature (CCBT) on the shoulder or on the wrist like a watch (Termdrop, Ava bracelet) or in the ear (YONO); the hiMAMA monitor works on a similar principle to iFertracker but has a lower purchase price and does not use disposable patches. Although they offer many additional measurements such as heart rate or respiratory rate, their reliability could be much discussed as they do not measure basal body core temperature. Their applicability is often limited to regular cycles (**Figure 6**).

3.5 OvuSense

OvuSense is a fully certified medical device, clinically proven in over 50,000 cycles of use. It measures core body temperature using a specially designed vaginal sensor, which is used overnight only, and data are downloaded to the dedicated OvuSense app each morning (**Figure 7**). OvuSense provides live updates

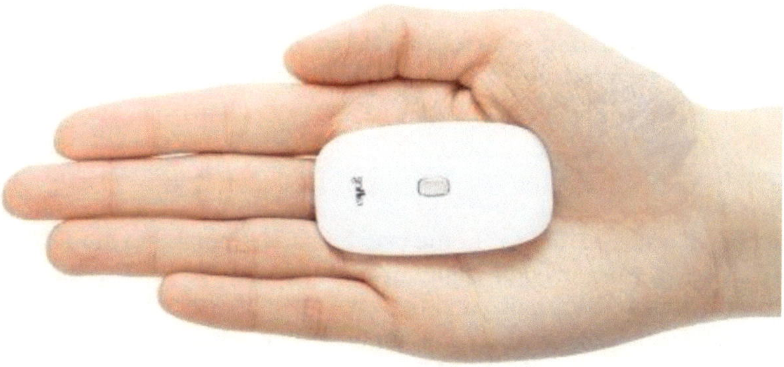

Figure 6.
iFertracker thermometer [15].

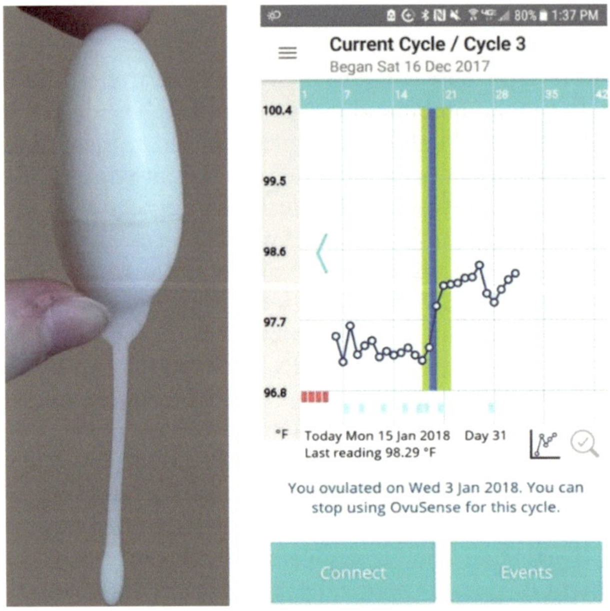

Figure 7.
OvuSense vaginal sensor and OvuSense app [17, 18].

predicting ovulation up to 24 hours in advance using current cycle data, then confirming the date of ovulation. At the start of each cycle, OvuSense provides a full 8-day fertile window. Vaginal sensor needs to be worn for a minimum of 4 hours during rest or sleep. It is essential to remove the sensor before using a bathroom or before going to have sex. OvuSense can be used alongside fertility medications and procedures; it has intelligent filtering systems that remove the temperature spikes outside of that range which is caused by illness or other exceptional situations. It is a class of medical device which is tested and conforms to strict medical standards. The sensor is made of antibacterial medical grade silicone, simply cleaned daily with warm water and soap. If the woman has completely regular ovulation, the live prediction has a positive predictive value of 96% and accurate ovulation confirmation of 99%. OvuSense Starter Pack 2-month subscription cost is $ 129 and its 1-year subscription cost is $ 210 [15, 16].

Another device which continuously collects body temperature from inside the body not only at night but during the day too is Priya—an intravaginal ring—as a fertility sensor. The ring measures the core body temperature every 6 min and sends the data wirelessly to a paired smartphone for monitoring and interpretation. The Priya Sensor is not yet available for sale. The limited release program started in late 2019 [17].

3.6 Persona

Persona is a diagnostic tool for home use. Persona records hormone levels (it measures the changes in estrogen-3-glucuronide (E3G) and luteinizing hormone (LH) concentrations) that accompany the ovulatory phase of the woman's menstrual cycle and considers the life span of sperm. The test stick captures hormones from morning urine, and the device then reads, records, and uses this information to tell you if you have a fertile day when you can get pregnant (a red light) or an infertile day when you cannot get pregnant (a green light) (**Figure 8**). The device determines 8 test days in each cycle, so the woman needs 8 test sticks (only in the

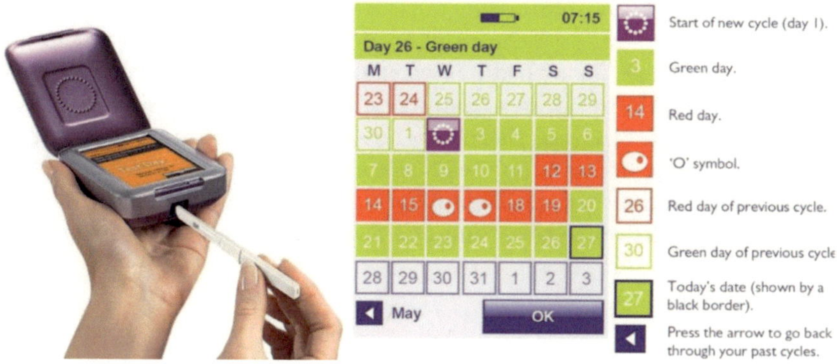

Figure 8.
Persona device and displayed data [18, 20].

first cycle the test is performed 16 times). Persona cannot be used by every woman, specifically women:

- Who cannot accept the possibility of pregnancy associated with the use of Persona (reliability confirmed by independent studies is 94%)
- With a cycle of less than 23 days
- With a cycle greater than 35 days
- Who have symptoms of menopause
- Who are breastfeeding
- Who use hormonal therapy, e.g., hormonal contraception, infertility treatment, hormone replacement therapy
- Who use any other treatment that affects their cycle
- Who use antibiotics containing tetracycline
- Who have reduced liver, kidney function, or polycystic ovary syndrome (PCOS) [18]

Persona is manufactured by SPD Swiss Precision Diagnostics GmbH in Switzerland. ClearBlue Easy Fertility monitor works on the same principle, but it is especially used to identify high-fertility days and achieve pregnancy. The price per Persona starts from $ 45; additional components or programs are not necessary, except for test sticks [19] (**Figure 8**).

4. Applications for natural family planning

The trends of the modern world are mobile applications; they are useful and easily available, and they can be used at any time with our mobile phone or tablet. The area of natural family planning did not also avoid the arrival of mobile applications. For the purpose of NFP, a lot of applications are available. Some offer reliable and quality results, but some are not recommended for use. However, all applications need input data, which are obtained by measuring basal body temperature, ovulation test result, or observation—the onset of menstruation, cervical mucus quality, etc. BBT can be measured by an ordinary thermometer with an accuracy of 0.01°C and enter values into the application manually. The second solution is measured values by digital Bluetooth basal thermometer—values are automatically written to the app when connected to a mobile phone, and the app also creates graphs, notifications, and statistical data. The following section will first describe wireless thermometers with custom applications and then stand-alone applications.

4.1 Cyclotest mySense

Cyclotest mySense is used to track the menstrual cycle without much effort, using Bluetooth technology. The basal temperature values measured each morning in 4-hour measuring window are transmitted wirelessly and directly to the smartphone. The thermometer is a Class IIb medical product, CE-certified, and thus approved for natural contraception. In the calculation of fertility, one of the observation data as cervical mucus quality or the result of an ovulation test (LH) can be included. The fertile phase is determined automatically in the application and offers a transparent view of the temperature curve and all additional inputs at all times. The application has two modes, fertility wish mode and contraception mode. The fertility algorithm is based on the symptothermal method and uses the algorithm of cyclotest myWay. The more recorded cycle the cyclotest mySense App has, the more accurate the forecast will be. If the measured temperature could be falsified by external influences, it should be excluded from the calculation directly in the application. Cyclotest mySense is suitable for cycles between 16 and 45 days, and the luteal phase should not be less than 11 days. The cyclotest mySense app is available for free, and the thermometer costs $ 122 (**Figure 9**).

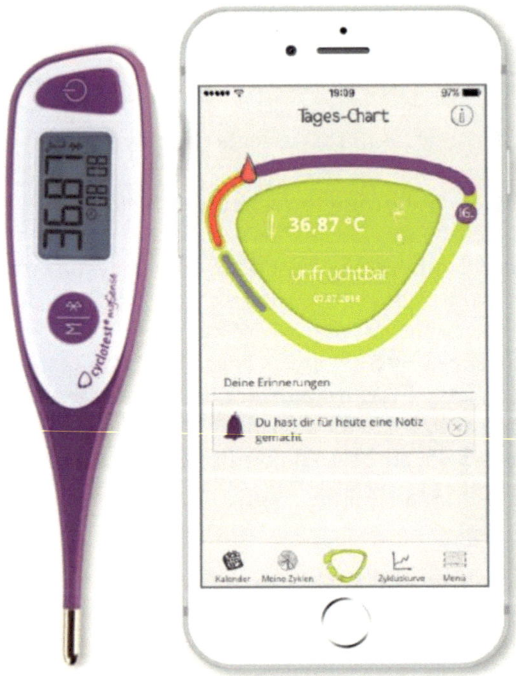

Figure 9.
Cyclotest mySense thermometer and app [21].

4.2 Biolight PregAid

Biolight basal thermometer is a device designed for daily temperature measurement and monitoring. The thermometer is able to store measured data and transfer it to PregAid application. The application is able to evaluate the measured data and thus determine fertile and infertile days, menstruation arrival even in an irregular cycle, or the possibility of pregnancy. This is ideal for women who are trying to conceive and have an irregular cycle. The thermometer is easy to use; just turn on the thermometer every morning after waking up, and measure the temperature under tongue for 3 minutes. By turning on the application, data will be saved and synchronized with the cloud. The cost of the device is $ 39.

The following products can also be included in the same user and price group of thermometers with own application as Biolight: Ovy, Kindara thermometer, TempCue, Femometer, PrecisionTemp, Xiaomi Mijia, and others.

4.3 Natural cycles

The natural birth control app uses a statistical algorithm that learns a woman's unique cycle from the BBT temperatures. Once Natural Cycles has analyzed the temperature curve, it can detect ovulation, learn fertile window, and determine the phase of the menstrual cycle. Natural Cycles offers a personalized fertility status every day. The application requires measurement of temperature at least 5 days a week within a 4-hour window. However, the fewer data are added, the more red days the app will give, hence recommending to use protection. Nature Cycles offers to add further data such as ovulation test results, premenstrual syndrome symptoms, and unprotected sex. The more data are put into the app, the more green days are going to get back. For irregularities as thyroid conditions, PCOS, or length of cycle out of range of 21–35 days, the app does not become any less effective. Natural Cycles is a handy tool for keeping track of irregularities in the cycle, but it gets more red days. The reliability declared by the manufacturer is 93% effective with typical use and 98% effective with perfect use (sexual abstinence or using condoms on red days).

Natural Cycles is in Europe the first CE-marked Class II medical device (CE0123) for use as a method of birth control, and in 2018 the US Food and Drug Administration (FDA) cleared Natural Cycles as a medical device for use as a digital method of birth control. The annual subscription (with thermometer) costs $ 71.76, and the monthly subscription costs $ 9.93 [22, 23].

4.4 OvuView

The application has no official website. Information can only be drawn from the Google Play Store and from the user experience or your own experience with the application.

OvuView offers three modes: (a) simple menstrual calendar, (b) achievement conception that highlights days with a high probability of pregnancy, and (c) preventing pregnancy. The app displays the menstrual wheel from which the day of the cycle, the number of days to menstruation, the start of fertile days, and the expected ovulation can be read, as well as the current phase of the cycle. Standard symptoms such as BBT and mucus symptoms are entered into the application. However, optional and intrinsic symptoms, e.g., mood, weight, PMS, and ovulation test can be recorded. When entering the observation of mucus, more symptoms of the predefined options can be selected at a time. Observation of mucus and the cervix is automatically rewritten into international symbols. The "Calendar" function displays clearly a calendar with evaluated and predicted values of menstruation and fertile days. The "Graph" function displays the temperature curve along with other recorded symptoms. OvuView evaluates symptoms based on the following rules:

- Rule 21/20 (six cycles recorded, no mucus)
- Döring rule (six recorded cycles, mucus)
- Rule B (temperature, mucus)
- Rule R (temperature, mucus)
- Rule K (temperature, mucus)
- Rule C or O (temperature, mucus)
- Rule of 5 dry days (mucus)
- Rule of four high temperatures (temperature)
- Rule of five high temperatures (temperature),
- Marshall rule (temperature)
- Last dry day rule (mucus, six cycles recorded, min. of 5-day long mucus episode)

Each method indicates what symptoms it needs for the evaluation, the rule's effectiveness, and the symbol, which indicates the phases can evaluate for a particular method. Each method can be switched on or off (e.g., a woman after taking a contraceptive can limit the evaluation only to the 5 T rule). The paid version costs $ 5 and offers extended functionalities: marking of low-temperature level and ovulation on the day when temperature increased; backup data to Google account (the free version can be backup to an SD card); sending data by e-mail and exporting graphs, password protection, widgets, own symptoms, alerts, e.g., mucus tracking, ovulation reminder, full picture mode, cycle management (pregnancy); removal of advertisements; and method selection/configuration.

To make the results as reliable as possible, OvuView offers the option to enter custom cycle lengths (longest and shortest) or to rely on general cycle lengths [24–28], which of course reduces reliability. If nothing is chosen, the application evaluates only based on the recorded cycles. Data can be imported from previously used another application.

According to the description on Google Play, the application evaluates using the symptothermal method as well as other methods. The description claims to be implementing 14 evaluating methods. In our opinion, this is a vague terminology, since the mentioned methods are actually the rules of the symptothermal method, of course, in addition to two trivial calendar calculation methods. However, it is not clear what precise didactic transposition of symptothermal method the app is. Compared to the paper form of evaluation, there are several differences in the electronic version. The reliability of the application depends on the accuracy and thoroughness of the entered data [29].

4.5 SymptoPlus

The SymptoPlus is not a medical device but an electronic learning tool to take charge of fertility. Application evaluation algorithm is based on a combination of three NFP methods—NFP-sensiplan (symptothermal method), Billings Ovulation Method (cervical mucus method), and Rötzer/Northwest Family Servis (NWFS, the American Rötzer version, symptothermal method). SymptoPlus is not an exactly didactic transposition of one particular method.

This stand-alone app doesn't require an Internet connection for its basic features. An Internet connection is only needed for syncing to secure access, even if losing the phone. To verify an account, go to sympto.org. After verifying an e-mail address, the 15 days free of charge of personal follow-up with a symptothermal expert without any commitment is available. After a 15-day trial, the SymptoPlus must be purchased in the Google Play Store for a nominal fee. A free version is also available, but SymptoPlus is faster and simpler to view than SymptoFree. The app is available in several languages and offers an internal message box which allows the client to communicate directly with her adviser.

For guaranteed contraceptive effectiveness, it is needed to use the app properly and use Sympto for 6 months with a counsellor (Daisy PLUS) or enter six past cycles verified by Sympto. To interpret a cycle correctly, Sympto has defined a minimum of 10 crucial information in order: the beginning of the cycle which is triggered by the 3 red drop icons, a minimum of 4 low temperatures within 6 days to specify the cover line, the mucus peak day indication (2 signs), and the 3 correct high temperatures [24, 25] (**Figure 10**).

The market offers a number of similar applications, e.g., myNFP, LilyPro, CycleProGo, Lady Cycle, etc. Some are more functional, others are less, and some can be used only as a record table without evaluating or with not reliable evaluating. The applications for NFP have a huge potential, but thorough research is needed. Medical doctor, developers, expert of didactic transpositions, learning specialists, teacher pairs for a specific method, and women using the app should work together

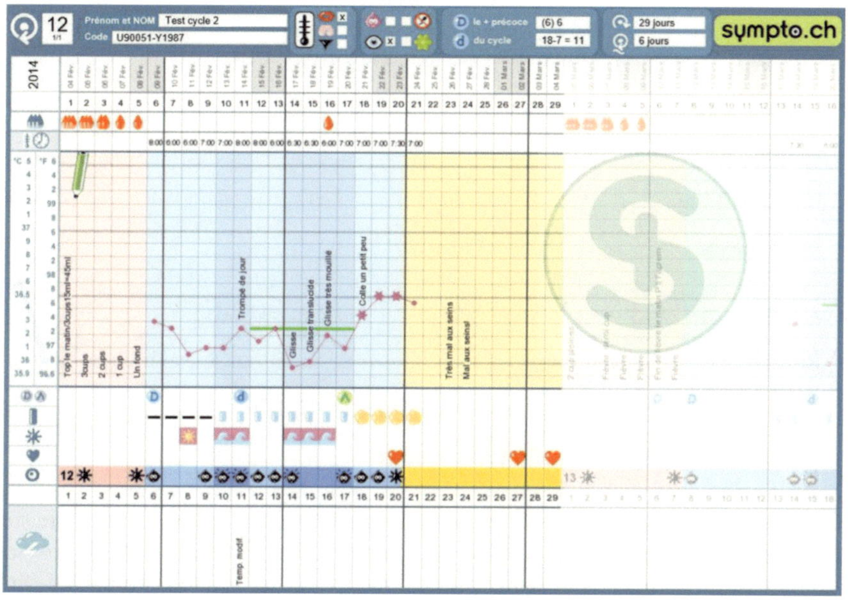

Figure 10.
SymptoPlus application record table [26].

to create the app. From this cooperation arise a quality application, which however must be subjected to in-depth testing on a sufficient number of cycles. Entered data must be accurate and obtained in accordance with the knowledge of symptothermal cycle observation.

5. SymRec

Applications and IT tools for NFP are an interesting research area, and based on how they were mentioned above, they have great potential. On the basis of these facts, we also decided to create a web site for evaluating the menstrual cycle according to symptothermal method (STM). The IT tool SymRec is an accurate didactic transposition of rules of STM used in Slovakia with some restriction listed below. We followed the rules outlined in the book *Handbook of Symptothermal Methods* published by Couple to Couple League in Slovakia [27].

The goal of the work was to create an IT tool—electronic record table (ERT)—similar to the printed record table used for symptothermal observation. ERT serves for daily data entry, storage data, and evaluating menstrual cycle according STM rules. Access to data is possible for every device connected to the Internet. ERT is available on the website: http://symrec.judak.eu/.

5.1 Didactic transposition of STM rules

Didactic transposition is the isolation of certain terms and properties from the environment in which they originated and their adaptation to the context in the new environment. In fact, it is the transfer of the regularities of the teaching or learning process (rules of some NFP method) from the analogue environment (manual paper method) to the digital environment (application, IT tool). It is an interpretation of NFP rules in the digital world using programming code. The original manual STM has been transformed into an electronic version by transcription to PHP code. ERT evaluates the record according to these rules:

1. Evaluation of the first phase of preovulatory infertility:
    - Last dry day rule
    - Doctors experience rule
    - Rule 20/21 days
    - Döring rule
2. Evaluation of the third phase of postovulatory infertility:
    - Rules R, B, and K—double-symptom rules (cervix mucus, basal body temperature)
    - 4 T, 5 T, and Marshall rule—one-symptom rules (BBT)
    - 5DMD—one-symptom rule (cervix mucus)

ERT expects that only valid temperatures are entered. Evaluation does not offer a possibility as "planning down" and averaging the temperatures, which are possible in manual evaluation in case of nonstandard temperature curves. To verify each rule, software checks at least six previous cycles and a maximum of thirteen cycles. According to the number of cycles in the recorded history of ERT, the evaluation is performed for the 8th recorded cycle, and a different evaluation rule is used for the

13th recorded cycle. It follows that for validation of all possibilities of evaluation, 27 rules have to be created. For evaluation of the first phase preovulatory infertility, it is necessary to have recorded at least six previous cycles—the STM rules require user experience with at least six previous cycles to allow for a reliable assessment of the current cycle. If there are not enough records in the recorded history of ERT, the evaluation for the first phase will not run, and the report with the alert to this situation is displayed.

The evaluation is possible until fulfilment at least one evaluation condition, e.g., for evaluation of the first phase, just enter the occurrence of cervical mucus, and the last dry day rule is activated. The accuracy of the evaluation depends on the amount of data collected, not only in the current cycle but also in previous cycles. The overall reliability of the ERT cannot be determined as the testing did not run with a statistically significant data set. As it is a precise didactic transposition of the rules and if accurate and clean data are entered, we assume reliability comparable to that of the symptothermal method. However, further testing with sufficient data is necessary to confirm this assumption.

6. Discussion

In this part of the paper, we discuss the problems associated with the use of NFP methods: the sense of using methods, determining reliability, and measuring basal body temperature.

The human body is an "unstable system," and when we talk about fertility, women respond very sensitively to various stimuli. Every organism is unique; no two cycles of the tens of thousands of observed cycles are identical. Due to the current rapid lifestyle, sedentary work, artificial lighting, or lack of physical exertion, menstrual cycle irregularities are more common than in the past, not to mention other reproductive health problems, e.g., polycystic ovary syndrome, myomas, pre-menstruation syndrome, etc. No device can predict in advance that there will be any irregularities in the current cycle that will shorten or extend the cycle. Nothing in the menstruation cycle can be predicted at a hundred percent. At the same time, there are periods in women's lives—e.g., before the first menstruation, after delivery, or in climacterium—when hormonal conditions can properly disrupt the cycle. From the experience of lecturers teaching NFP methods, it can be argued that in these cases the devices or applications cannot reliably evaluate the course of the cycle and pairs have to rely on prolonged sexual abstinence or use of barrier contraception due to inaccurate device estimation.

The accuracy of the outputs of the technical aids depends not only on the quality of the components they are made of but also on the software that makes the evaluation itself. Even the finest instruments and the most sophisticated software for determining fertile and infertile days have their limits, and it is not good to rely blindly on them. Even those who welcome technical innovations are advised to supplement the information from the device with their personal assessment of fertility symptoms (at least one symptom). Users will avoid unnecessary disappointment from possible failure, especially during nonstandard situations. Learning to understand some NFP methods is not as difficult as it may seem. Indeed, one of the prerequisites of NFP methods is knowing your own body, not mechanically thoughtless entering data into device/application.

The determination of the reliability of NFP methods can have a discussion for a long time. It is difficult to determine the evaluation criteria that will deliver the most relevant results. The most commonly used Pearl Index (PI) is under criticism because of the fact that different PI values are found in the literature for one method [30]. Key parameters that are subject to comparability should be used to calculate the reliability of the method:

a. Frequency of sexual intercourse—the difference is in recording 1 unwanted pregnancy for 5 years at 1 intercourse as 1 pregnancy for 5 years at 300 (or more) intercourses.

b. Sample size—no sample size is specified for PI determination. The larger the sample, the more accurate the result.

c. Age of women—fertility is different at every woman's age. The chance to conceive naturally in a 20-year-old woman is significantly higher than in a 38-year-old woman. Also, men's fertility rates decline by age [31].

d. The period of application of the method—unexpected pregnancies usually come in the first months of using a particular method. The longer the couples use the method, the more they are trained, and the number of unexpected pregnancies decreases.

e. User error—if an unexpected pregnancy occurs as a result of a conscious mistake by the user (e.g., situations where the partners have sexual intercourse during a period they know is fertile or use a barrier contraception during the fertile period), this situation should be recorded and should not be taken into account in establishing rate reliability.

f. BMI—overweight and obese women have a significant relationship between body mass index, spotting, menstrual cycle length, menstrual bleeding, and passing clots [30].

g. Diseases/medicaments/residual contraceptives.

A certain solution is to determine the reliability of typical use and perfect use, but the criteria mentioned above must be considered in this case too. Either, the individual approach of women to the use of a particular method should not be forgotten. Every woman is different; there is no universal solution for all women; however, solutions can be found for groups with similar method requirements. It is worth reminding that none of the NFP methods is 100% reliable (perfect use). In preventing unplanned pregnancy, only three methods of conceiving regulation have 100% reliability:

- 100% sexual abstinence (no genital contact).
- Removal of both testes.
- Removal of both ovaries.

All other methods of conceiving control have some degrees of failure. Failures of NFP, e.g., symptothermal method, in the most cases are caused by inconsistent observation and recording of fertility symptoms, the use of barrier methods in the fertile phase of the cycle, and the conscious reliance on chance [27].

The basal temperature measurement time frame is a topic that we supposedly should be giving due consideration too. Basal body temperature assessment is well described and applied. However, the time range of basal temperature measuring remains a problem. This range is differently set for devices (Cyclotest myWay ±2 hours, Lady-Comp ±3 hours, Daysy no timeframe) and applications (Cyclotest mySense ±2 hours, Natural Cycles ±2 hours). Of course, this problem is eliminated in continuous temperature monitoring (iFertracker, OvuSense), although a system for determining a particular temperature, e.g., from 100 measured values, can be discussed. The question remains how much are the objective results of the measured basal temperature in an interval of 6 hours. Under normal circumstances, BBT reaches its lowest in the early morning hours and then rises by about 0.05°C every half hour. Thus, the BBT measured outside the tolerated range of 30 minutes may not be accurate. Dr. Rötzer states in his work that basal temperatures measured outside the tolerance range (±30 minutes) after 7:30 am tend to have a greater effect on the temperature curve than deviations measured in the early morning hours [32]. So wide time frame is naturally comfortable for users, but the most accurate results can be achieved by measuring at the same time every day. The condition of daily measurement also plays an important role in the degree of reliability.

The task of experts is to find a solution in the field of NFP that confirms the words by Will Sacks, which aptly described the present state of fertility control with words: "I think the last century was about solving health problems with pills and synthetics, and this century is about solving health problems with software and data. The pill was an enormous boon for the previous generation. It set women free in so many ways, but it also came with side effects that a lot of women nowadays are finding unacceptable. Fertility Awareness is effective, low-cost, and side-effect-free so I think women and couples are finding it an attractive option. I also happen to think that Fertility Awareness is a consciousness-raising tool—it helps women tune into and feel powerful and in control of their health, and it helps male partners better understand the feminine. As consciousness and mindfulness increase globally, using synthetic hormones to control fertility is becoming less acceptable, and Fertility Awareness, which is the practice of living in harmony with your cycle, is becoming more obvious" [33].

7. Conclusion

The paper provides an overview of technical devices and applications used for evaluating the menstrual cycle and determining fertile and infertile days. In the first part, the principle of using and evaluating the four most commonly used NFP methods is briefly described. The next part is devoted to currently available information technologies and electronic devices designed to evaluate the menstrual cycle in terms of NFP methods. The conditions of use, reliability, price, and limitations for the six devices and five applications are described. Finally, our proposed system of fertility assessment based on STM in the form of a website is described. The discussion critically evaluates the possibilities of use and weaknesses of the described technical devices and information means.

It follows that the success of the use of electronic devices or applications needs to be strengthened by some degree of knowledge and experience in assessing self-fertility. Although manufacturers report high reliability of their products, there is no need to blindly rely on the device and application results and evaluation should be complemented with own judgment. For a successful creation of quality and reliable application or device, cooperation from experts in various fields of science is needed, and research and experiences of practical users is necessary.

Author details

Zuzana Judáková
Faculty of Electrical Engineering and Information Technology, Department of Electromagnetic and Biomedical Engineering, University of Žilina, Žilina, Slovak Republic

*Address all correspondence to: zuzana.judakova@feit.uniza.sk

References

[1] World Health Organization. Natural Family Planning: A Guide to Provision of Services. Switzerland: Geneva; 1988. p. 92

[2] Indian Council of Medical Research Task Force on Natural Family Planning. Field trial of billings ovulation method of natural family planning. Contraception. 1996;**53**:69-74

[3] Händel P, Wahlström J. Digital contraceptives based on basal body temperature measurements. Biomedical Signal Processing and Control. 2019;**52**:141-151. DOI: 10.1016/j.bspc.2019.04.019

[4] Rötzer J. Erweiterte Basaltemperaturmessung und Empfängnisregelung. Archiv für Gynäkologie. 1968;**205**(2):195-214

[5] Frank-Herrmann P, Gnoth C, Toledo E, Baur S, Pyper C, Jenetzky E, et al. The effectiveness of a fertility awareness based method to avoid pregnancy in relation to a couple's sexual behaviour during the fertile time: A prospective longitudinal study. Human Reproduction. 2007;**22**(5):1310-1319

[6] Frank-Herrmann P, Sottong U, Baur S, Raith-Paula E, Strowitzki T, Freundl G. Natürliche Familienplanung: Sensiplan®—eine moderne, verlässliche Methode. Der Gynäkologe. 2011;**44**(1):17-22

[7] Kambic RT, Lamprecht V. Calendar rhythm efficacy: A review. Advances in Contraception. 1996;**12**(2):123-128

[8] UEBE Medical GmbH. Online-Shop [Internet]. 2019. Available from: https://www.cyclotest.de/produkte/

[9] Freundl G, Frank-Herrmann P, Godehardt E, Klemm R, Bachhofer M. Retrospective clinical trial of contraceptive effectiveness of the electronic fertility indicator Ladycomp/Babycomp. Advances in Contraception. 1988;**14**:98-108

[10] Come Correggere la Data su Lady-Comp o Pearly [Internet]. 2019. Available from: https://blog.babycomp.it/correggere_la_data_ladycomp_pearly/

[11] Valley Electronics LLC. Lady Comp ovulation calculator [Internet]. 2019. Available from: https://lady-comp.com/

[12] Valley Electronics AG. Daysy fertility tracker [Internet]. 2019. Available from: https://daysy.me/

[13] Valley Electronics. Daysy fertility monitor [Internet]. 2019. Available from: https://www.stressnomore.co.uk/valley-electronics-daysy-fertility-monitor-11246.html

[14] Raiing Medical Company. The Smart Fertility Tracker–iFertracker [Internet]. 2019. Available from: https://ifertracker.com/

[15] Papaioannou S, Delkos D, Pardey J, Milnes RC, Knowles TG. Vaginal core body temperature assessment identifies pre-ovulatory body temperature rise and detects ovulation in advance of ultrasound folliculometry. Human Reproduction. 2014;**29**:219-220

[16] Fertility Focus Inc. OvuSense [Internet]. 2019. Available from: https://www.ovusense.com/

[17] The Priya Sensor. Prima-Temp [Internet]. 2019. Available from: http://www.prima-temp.com/solutions

[18] Hormone Free Contraception. PERSONA manual [Internet]. 2019. Available from: https://cdn2.clearblue.com/sites/default/files/wysiwyg/leaflets/2300406_02_english.pdf

[19] Persona Contraception Monitor. 1 Touch Screen Monitor: Amazon, Health

& Personal Care [Internet]. 2019. Available from: https://www.amazon.co.uk/Persona-Contraception-Monitor-Touch-Screen/dp/B01B0OB79W/ref=pd_bxgy_img_2

[20] Persona Contraception Monitor | Home Health UK [Internet]. 2019. Available from: https://homehealth-uk.com/all-products/advanced-persona-ovulation-contraception-monitor/

[21] Cyclotest mySense Bluetooth-Thermometer [Internet]. 2019. Available from: https://www.cyclotest.de/cyclotest-mysense/

[22] Natural Cycles. Contraceptive Methods [Internet]. 2019. Available from: https://www.naturalcycles.com/birthcontrol/is-natural-cycles-for-me/

[23] Berglund Scherwitzl E, Lundberg O, Kopp Kallner H, Gemzell Danielsson K, Trussell J, Scherwitzl R. Perfect-use and typical-use Pearl Index of a contraceptive mobile app. Contraception. 2017;**96**(6):420-425. DOI: 10.1016/j.contraception.2017.08.014

[24] Sympto—The natural management of your fertility, online and on mobile phone [Internet]. 2019. Available from: http://www.sympto.ch/technique_en.html

[25] Ducamp M, Lotrea A. Symptothermal contraception with smartphone apps [Internet]. 2014. Available from: https://sympto.org/3/en/full-comparative-app-study-of-2014

[26] SymptoPlus record 12 [Internet]. Available from: https://sympto.org/3/en/full-comparative-app-study-of-2014

[27] Predáč J, Predáčová S. Handbook of Symptothermal Methods NFP and Ecological Breastfeeding. 3rd ed. Olomouc: Liga pár páru v Slovenskej republike; 2014. pp. 181. Available from: https://www.lpp.sk/ponuka/produkt/7-prirucka-stm-ppr

[28] Trussell J, Portman D. The creeping pearl: Why has the rate of contraceptive failure increased in clinical trials of combined hormonal contraceptive pills? Contraception. 2013;**88**(5):604-610. DOI: 10.1016/j.contraception.2013.04.001

[29] Apps on Google Play: OvuView [Internet]. 2019. Available from: https://play.google.com/store/apps/details?id=com.sleekbit.ovuview

[30] Tayebi N, Yazdanpanahi Z, Yektatalab S, Pourahmad S, Akbarzadeh M. The relationship between body mass index (BMI) and menstrual disorders at different ages of menarche and sex hormones. Journal of the National Medical Association. 2018;**110**(5):440-447. DOI: 10.1016/j.jnma.2017.10.007

[31] Dunson DB, Baird DD, Colombo B. Increased infertility with age in men and women. Obstetrics and Gynecology. 2004;**103**(1):51-56

[32] Rötzer J, Rötzer E. Natürliche Empfängnisregelung—Der partnerschaftliche Weg—Die sympto-thermale Methode. Basel, Wien: Freiburg; 2003. pp. 143

[33] Wink by Kindara: Fertility Awareness Made Simple, Ladyclever [Internet]. 2019. Available from: https://ladyclever.com/health-fitness/wink-by-kindara-fertility-awareness-made-simple/

Section 3

Family Planning Practices in Developing Countries

Chapter 3

Reproductive Health and Family Planning Services in Africa: Looking beyond Individual and Household Factors

Alhaji A. Aliyu and Tukur Dahiru

Abstract

Worldwide, there have been remarkable gains in the provision and utilization of reproductive health and FP services. However, in Africa, despite increasing availability, utilization of these services is less than 50%, even though there are wide variations among and within the countries across the continent. Articles from peer-reviewed journals, technical reports, Internet articles, grey literature (official government documents, technical reports, etc.) and Demographic and Health Survey (DHS) reports were used as resource materials. Manual search of reference list of selected articles was done for further relevant materials. We also used for comparative analysis, the online StatCompiler tool (https://www.statcompiler.com/en/) to extract data. Reproductive health and contraceptives have a lot of benefits to the individual, family and community. However, despite near universal knowledge and availability of reproductive health and FP services in Africa, utilization of these services is less than optimal. Several factors operating at individual, household and within the community influence utilization of services. These factors are the cause of poor maternal health and care that might hinder population health and the attainment of Sustainable Development Goals (SDGs). Interventions to promote and sustain utilization of services should target these factors at different levels depending upon relative role/s of these factors.

Keywords: antenatal care, facility delivery, skilled attendant, postnatal care, FP, service utilization, SSA

1. Introduction

Inequality in health care utilization and large disparities in health outcomes exists between countries and even within them. These differences largely are defined and perpetrated by a multitude of factors-social structures-and mediated by material and behavioral factors and by aspects of health system delivery [1]. Thirty years after the launch of Safe Motherhood Initiative, the health and well-being of mothers and newborns have improved appreciably in many countries. However, countries with the highest burdens of mortality and illness have made least progress and inequalities between countries are increasing. Worldwide, each year, there are about 3.2 million stillborn babies, 4 million neonatal deaths and

0.5 million maternal deaths [2]. In majority of situations, the deaths are largely preventable [2, 3]. Around 99% of these deaths occurs in developing countries [2] out of which 11–17% of maternal deaths occurs during childbirth and 50–71% of it in the postpartum period [4]. While every pregnancy carries risks [4, 5] that must be addressed by skilled health providers, the timing, spacing and above all, the women's ability to decide when to become pregnant are key to favorable pregnancy outcomes.

Sexual and reproductive health (SRH) is a relatively new concept in the context of the dynamics of contemporary public health issues. It is closely related to the trio of health, population and environment (PHE), the three topmost challenging issues that require global attention for solutions. SRH is significantly influenced by socio-cultural, political and religious considerations [6, 7]. The five core components of sexual and reproductive health include among others improvement of antenatal, postnatal, postpartum and newborn care, provision of high-quality services including family planning (FP), etc. Pregnancy is a physiological process of activities in a continuum, each activity (or stage) crucially influenced by the preceding activity (or stage).

It is well recognized that improving the women's chances of surviving pregnancy and child birth relies on their access to reproductive health including FP. And within the continuum of maternity care, antenatal care (ANC) provides an avenue for important health care functions such as health education, health promotion, screening and diagnosis and disease prevention [8]. Studies have reported that ANC alone can reduce maternal mortality by up to 20%, given good quality and regular attendance [4, 9]. Maternal health care services in developing countries have evolved rather slowly. The first intervention to be implemented in a widespread fashion within maternal health programs was antenatal care. Delivery care (either institutional or home-based) was a later addition [10], while systematic and regular postpartum follow-up and care are hardly available [11]. Poor maternal health thus remains a major reproductive health concern in most part of the developing nations including SSA. Relatively less progress has been made in the area of maternal health compared to the reductions in fertility and infant mortality [12]. It has been estimated that in 2009, the lifetime risk of maternal death in SSA was 1 in 16 (compared to 1 in 2800 in developed regions) and that maternal mortality ratios were 540 in Ghana, 1000 in Kenya, 800 in Nigeria and 880 in Uganda, respectively [13, 14]. The sad reality of the situation is that these deaths can be prevented by simple and cost-effective public health interventions such as giving pregnant women tetanus toxoid injections together with other antenatal care services as well as postnatal care. Because women comprise more than half of the total population of most SSA countries, poor maternal health and care can be a huge obstacle to human and sustainable socio-economic development.

Access to reproductive health services is skewed in favor of urban areas to the detriment of the majority of rural population. Studies have shown how socio-economic, socio-cultural variables and demographics influenced the demand for and utilization of maternal and child health services [15–17]. For instance, maternal education has been found to be a significant predictor of the use of maternal health care services [18, 19]. Additionally, the costs [20], location [21, 22] and quality of health services are also important. Predictably, these factors interact in different ways to determine the use of health care. Thus, many women in SSA have unmet need for contraceptive and reproductive health services. Unmet reproductive health needs exist if there is a gap between a perceived need and the current available options to satisfy the need [23].

Family planning (FP) for the purpose of child spacing is not alien to African culture. Traditionally, African mothers practice intensive breastfeeding lasting longer than 24 months (and in some cultures up to 36 months). Some African societies practice postpartum marital sexual separation where the woman spends most of the postpartum period with her parents receiving special traditional and cultural rites for health and vitality [24]. This long period of voluntary separation ensures that sexual intercourse does not happen to avoid pregnancy. However, modern family planning programs, that is, organized effort to provide contraception to women and men, appeared on the sub-continent in 1950s. During the 1950s, there were attempts to establish family planning programs across the region. First, it was in Rhodesia in 1955, then Uganda in 1956, then Kenya in 1957, Mauritius in 1957, Nigeria in 1958 and Sierra Leone in 1959 [25]. By mid-1960s, family planning clinics were scattered across some of these countries offering family planning commodities. Thus, family planning clinics sprang up in the major cities such as Salisbury (Zimbabwe), Nairobi (Kenya), Kampala (Uganda), Lagos and Ibadan (Nigeria), Freetown (Liberia) and Accra (Ghana). Though these family planning clinics were established either by the government or by private associations, there was vehement resistance coming from both the religious and cultural institutions. The landscape remained the same well into 1970s with many countries in this region showing lackadaisical attitudes toward expansion of the services, with quite a handful of these governments indicating that they are not worried about the rate of population growth. However, this position began to change by early 1980s with a global economic meltdown and these governments actively saw the need to intervene to bring down fertility rate via vigorous family planning programs. Since a woman's overall reproductive health is determined collectively by the overall coverage, context, quality and utilization, it is important to assess the levels, trends and barriers of service utilization. Understanding the determinants that affect the utilization of these important reproductive health and FP services can assist in developing policies and designing interventions aimed at improving service utilization in countries across SSA. This will go a long way in reducing maternal mortality.

2. Reproductive health: antenatal care

Antenatal care (ANC) basically means care before birth. The aim of ANC is to assist pregnant women to remain healthy, finding and correcting adverse conditions when present and aiding the health of the unborn baby [26]. Within the continuum of maternity care, ANC provides a platform for critical health care functions. These include health promotion, screening and diagnosis and disease prevention [8]. Studies have reported that ANC alone can reduce maternal mortality by 20% with regular attendance and of good quality [4, 9]. Research has shown that achieving the World Health Organization (WHO) recommended four individualized ANC visits at 90% coverage rate could save about 37–71% [27] of newborn deaths, and 67% of death of newborns in SSA could be prevented by high average of care [28]. It also provides an avenue for encouraging skilled attendance at birth [29], early detection and management of potential complications [30] and provision of health education on good nutrition, family planning and breastfeeding [31, 32]. ANC during pregnancy has a positive influence on the utilization of postnatal health care services. The developed world has achieved remarkable success in ANC coverage with over 80% of woman having at least one ANC visit. However, many countries in SSA still have less impressive levels below the WHO recommended four or more visits. In most situations, the women in SSA wait till second or third trimester to make the initial ANC visit, thereby reducing the chances of making at least four visits [32, 33].

Several studies have assessed individual and household determinants in the utilization of reproductive health services in SSA. For instance, socio-demographic, religion, accessibility, educational status and affordability (socio-economic status) [12, 34–38] were all found to determine antenatal care utilization. The influence of these factors varied between countries across the continent. In Zimbabwe, poor quality of care and attitudes of service providers were barriers to utilization of services [39]. It can be assumed that utilization of maternal health services depends not only on individual and household factors but also importantly within the context of the country where the individual resides. Understanding this context is the key to improving service utilization since the individuals or couples are nested with families, which are in turn nested within communities. Studies have shown that family and community membership constitutes a major determinant in access to ANC services [27, 40].

3. Health facility delivery and skilled attendant at birth

While motherhood is often a positive and fulfilling experience, for too many women, it is associated with suffering, pain, ill-health and even death. Delivery at a health facility with assistance of skilled medical professional reduces the risk of complications and infections during labor and delivery. Skilled birth attendance is the process by which a woman is provided adequate care by trained health personnel during labor, delivery and early postnatal period. It is the single most cost-effective intervention in reducing maternal and perinatal mortality. In the developing countries, one third of all pregnant women receive no health talk, 60% of all deliveries take place outside health care facilities and about 46.7% of all deliveries are attended to by trained health personnel [41, 42]. Epidemiologic data on maternal deaths in developing countries revealed that two-thirds of death occur around the time of delivery [43]. Obstetric complication can occur around the time of delivery and cannot be predicted. Thus, it is important that all pregnant women have access to a skilled attendant to manage normal delivery and who can also recognize and manage obstetric complications or refer to high-level facility when necessary.

Across the continent, variations exist at individual, household and community contexts on the factors that influence the utilization of these services. Several individual factors that affect the use of ANC significantly influence the use of skilled personnel for delivery. Skilled attendance at delivery is an important factor in preventing maternal deaths and it is also crucial to prevent stillbirths and improve newborn survival [44, 45]. There are wide variations across SSA on health facility delivery and birth attended to by skilled personnel. In Nigeria, health facility delivery (39%) and skilled attendant at delivery (43%) are very low [46]. While in Zimbabwe, 77% of births took place in health facility and about 8 in 10 deliveries are assisted by a skilled provider (majority by a nurse or nurse midwife, 66%) [47]. There has been a progressive remarkable improvement in Ghana, where facility delivery increased from 54% in 2007 to 79% in 2017 and skilled attendant at delivery was 79% [48]. According to recent demographic and health survey (DHS), facility delivery and skilled attendant in Tanzania were respectively 63% and 64% [49]. Previous studies have shown consistent association between urban residence and utilization of ANC, delivery and PNC services [50]. In general, the decisions that lead women to use services seem to reside within the context of their marriage. Since individuals and families all live within the community, it definitely can influence personal health–seeking behavior as there are personnel beliefs and attitudes and community norms [51]. Again, religion and to a large extent ethnicity often influence beliefs, norms and values in relation to pregnancy, childbirth and utilization of services [44, 50]. The variations in factors and diversity within the populations of women could be explained by differences in women's autonomy, empowerment, gender relationships and social networks, which are in turn influenced by embedded social structures, religion and cultural beliefs. For instance, non-white South African women usually attend ANC later in pregnancy because it is viewed as being necessary to allow access to facility delivery [52].

Even though ANC is universally free in most countries in SSA, this does not translate into use of skilled attendance at delivery, since less than 50% of all women are assisted by skilled professional during delivery. SSA is the region with the lowest coverage of skilled delivery utilization with only 45% of women having skilled attendants at birth [50]. From a country-specific context, there are wide variations across and within the countries across the continent, with 10% skilled delivery utilization in Ethiopia [53], 43% in Nigeria [46] to 52% in Kenya [54].

About half of postpartum deaths take place within one day of delivery and roughly 70% occur within the first week. Obviously, there is mismatch between women's need for reproductive health care and what is currently available in terms of its provision and service utilization across SSA. Large body of evidence on factors contributing to poor service utilization consistently showed physical and financial barriers as well as educational level, parity, residence, ANC attendance and social status of the women [50, 55–58]. Expectedly, better educated women and those who had better autonomy in decisions pertaining to household expenses were more likely to have facility delivery [55]. In the context of achieving universal health coverage through improving health systems strengthening, barriers still remain in the utilization of reproductive health services.

4. Postnatal care (PNC)

Worldwide, about half of maternal deaths occur within the first 24 h after delivery. WHO guidelines that most countries in SSA adopted recommends that women who deliver in a health facility receive postnatal care check in the 24 h after delivery, while those who gave birth outside a health facility should be referred for postnatal checks in health facility within 12 h after delivery. PNC is part of continuum of care started from ANC. Thus, antenatal care promotes the use of PNC services for the mother-child pair [33]. As a major component of PNC, immunization remains to be one of the most effective public health interventions that have been proven to prevent about 24% of the 10 million deaths of children under five years annually [59]. Postnatal care (PNC) is one of the recommended strategies to reduce maternal and newborn deaths during the postpartum period [27, 60]. It is further recommended that mothers and newborns receive PNC in health facilities for at least 24 h after birth for those who delivered in the facility. While for those who delivered outside the health facility (at home), the first postnatal contact should be within 24 h of birth. At least 3 additional postnatal contacts are recommended for both mothers and newborns on day 3 (48–72 h), between days 7 and 14 after birth and 6 weeks after birth [61]. As with other maternal health services, PNC utilization is weak or low in SSA among all reproductive and child health programs. PNC utilization in Ethiopia is very low with only 7.1% of women [50] having PNC service in the first 2 days after delivery, 42% in Nigeria [46], 57% in Zimbabwe [47], 12.8% in Rwanda [62], 31% in Tanzania [63] and 58% in Uganda [64], respectively.

Again, physical accessibility is one of the most important variables in health service utilization. Several studies have shown that proximity of health care services play an important role in service utilization [21, 50, 65]. A number of individual, household and institutional characteristics affect women's decision in seeking health care. In general, despite the availability of reproductive health services, the decisions that lead women to use the services resides within the context of their marriage, household and family/community settings. The use of ANC during pregnancy is a major predictor of subsequent use of skilled delivery and PNC services. Therefore, the importance of ANC utilization as a key entry point to increase PNC services cannot be overemphasized. The early postpartum period can be targeted as the best period to discuss FP methods with the couples.

5. Family planning: levels of knowledge of contraceptive methods

Knowledge of at least any modern method among the women is almost universal across the countries (**Table 1**). The earliest information on knowledge of any modern method of contraception is the Nigeria Demographic and Health Survey (DHS) of 1990 and it reported a level of 41.2%, which coincidentally is lowest among the countries, while Burundi reported the highest level of 99.2% in 2016–2017 [66]. The level of knowledge varied markedly among countries with lowest knowledge level of 63.5% reported from Chad DHS of 2014–2015 to the highest (universal) of 100% in Rwanda [66]. In terms of percent change, Comoros recorded the smallest change in knowledge of 0.4%, while Nigeria recorded the highest of 52.7%.

5.1 Levels and trends of ever use of modern contraception

The level and trend in ever use of modern contraception among the women was reported by 24 countries; many other countries did not collect this information between surveys. Ever use of modern contraception was lowest in Chad, 2.8% (1996/1997 survey) and 5.2% in most recent survey (2004) while Zimbabwe had the highest levels of 85.2% (2005/2006 survey) [47], respectively. Malawi recorded the greatest change (increase) in ever use of modern contraception of 55.4%. There has always being a great gap between knowledge and practice (ever use) of modern contraception particularly in sub-Saharan Africa (**Figure 1**) [67]. The difference between knowledge and ever use of a modern method of contraception is widest in Niger (77.6%) and narrowest in Zimbabwe (14.5%). This is not surprising as Niger Republic is traditionally a high-fertility country coupled with low literacy level, strong cultural and religious opposition to modern contraception and early age at marriage. However, the story is different with Zimbabwe often cited as one of the few success stories in sub-Saharan Africa where family planning services appeared in the country as far back as 1953 coupled with cultural and religious tolerance to its use [68].

5.2 Levels and trends of current use of modern contraception

Current use of modern contraception among countries in SSA showed variability with Chad having the lowest of 5.0%, while Zimbabwe had the highest at 65.8%. Two countries, Liberia and Senegal, had their earliest DHS to have been conducted in 1986, which showed a very low uptake of modern contraception at 5.5% and 2.1%, respectively. South Africa conducted its earliest DHS in 1998 with an uptake of modern contraception of 55.1%; the same country that conducted its recent DHS in 2016 reported a decline in uptake to 54.0% (or a drop of 1.1%). Malawi recorded the greatest change between its earliest and most recent survey of 50.7% [66]. Again, the greatest disparity between knowledge and current use of modern contraception is as shown in **Figure 2**. Across the globe, this pattern has been reported particularly in developing countries [68].

	Country	Earliest	Recent	Change
1	Benin	76.2	96.3	20.1
2	Burkina Faso	63.3	97.5	34.2
3	Burundi	99.2	99.7	0.5
4	Cameroon	62.9	94.0	31.1
5	Chad	42.8	63.5	20.7
6	Comoros	98.1	98.5	0.4
7	Congo	96.3	98.6	2.3
8	Congo Democratic Republic	76.7	89.9	13.2
9	Cote d'Ivoire	71.5	93.2	21.7
10	Eritrea	62.0	87.2	25.2
11	Ethiopia	85.3	98.7	13.4
12	Gabon	94.7	97.6	2.9
13	Ghana	90.7	99.2	8.5
14	Guinea	69.1	84.8	15.7
15	Kenya	96.9	98.7	1.8
16	Lesotho	98.1	99.5	1.4
17	Liberia	86.7	98.6	11.9
18	Madagascar	61.7	95.0	33.3
19	Malawi	91.8	99.6	7.8
20	Mali	64.6	94.4	29.8
21	Mozambique	60.4	96.3	35.9
22	Namibia	90.3	99.8	9.5
23	Niger	58.0	89.3	31.3
24	Nigeria	41.2	93.9	52.7
25	Rwanda	96.8	100.0	3.2
26	Senegal	70.4	97.2	26.8
27	Sierra Leone	66.2	93.7	27.5
28	South Africa	98.0	99.9	1.9
29	Tanzania	77.6	99.1	21.5
30	Togo	93.4	97.1	3.7
31	Uganda	91.6	99.7	8.1
32	Zambia	90.7	99.7	9.0
33	Zimbabwe	98.5	99.7	1.2

Table 1.
Percentage of currently married women who know any modern method of contraception, DHS surveys 1990–2018 [66].

5.3 Sources of modern contraceptive methods

It is generally believed that as the demand for modern contraception increases, the supply as well as outlets will increase and at the same time become diversified [67]. Initially, modern contraception is almost solely provided by government through its formal outlets such as hospitals, family planning clinics, health clinics,

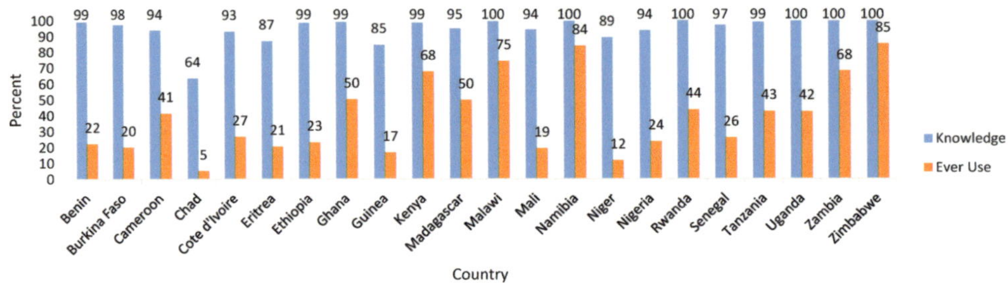

Figure 1.
Gap between knowledge and ever use of modern contraception, DHS surveys [66].

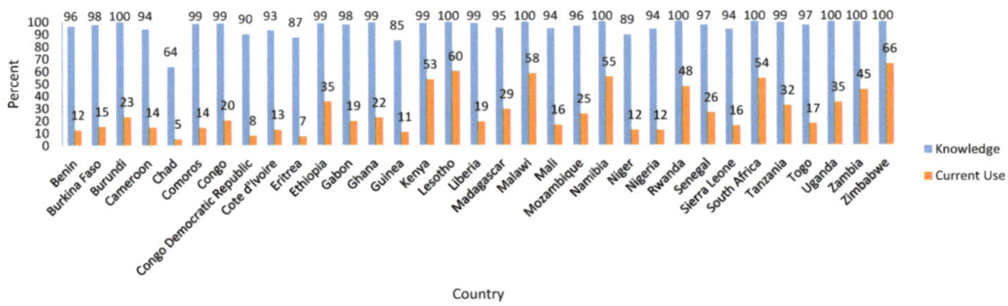

Figure 2.
Gap between knowledge and current use of modern contraception, DHS surveys [66].

etc. However, with an increase in demand and acceptance, the sources began to expand and more providers appeared in the market such as private non-governmental organizations and religious and faith-based organizations (**Table 2**). Across sub-Saharan Africa, public outlet is the predominant as well as important source of information on contraception. This is not surprising because of the misconceptions associated with it. It is much later that private medical outlets and then other private non-medical outlets joined the supply and service outlet.

Marked variability exists across the continent on public source as supplier of contraceptive commodity accounting for 20.7% in Democratic Republic of Congo, 91.3% Rwanda and 93.3% Niger, respectively [66]. Regarding the changes in the proportion of public source of information and contraception, Uganda and Madagascar recorded the greatest changes. There was a decline in Uganda, while Madagascar recorded an increase in the role of public outlet of contraception. The reasons for this might be due to influx of other non-public (or governmental) supplies or a decline in quality of services as well as supply of the commodity. For those that recorded an increase in this proportion, probably the government in recent times is becoming more active in FP programs. Decline in the proportion of women obtaining information and contraception from public outlet has been documented earlier [67]. In this analysis, 12 countries (or 38%) experienced a decline in the percentage of women getting contraception from public channels, while in the remaining countries, it increased. Thus, it is reasonable to assume that an expansion of high-quality services might increase women's motivation to use these services.

5.4 Contraceptive discontinuation and switching

There are several reasons why a woman currently using a modern contraception would discontinue or switch to another method. Some of these reasons could be health-related such as experiencing intolerable side effects (hypertension, obesity, etc.). More often, it is fertility-related such as a desire to become pregnant, or it

	Country	Earliest	Recent	Change
1	Benin	43.5	62.4	18.9
2	Burkina Faso	64.6	73.7	9.1
3	Burundi	87.3	80.9	-6.4
4	Cameroon	30.5	20.0	-10.5
5	Chad	59.3	71.6	12.3
6	Comoros	77.6	87.2	9.6
7	Congo	22.0	19.4	-2.6
8	Congo Democratic Republic	20.7	31.1	10.4
9	Cote d'Ivoire	25.5	26.3	0.8
10	Eritrea	78.4	74.0	-4.4
11	Ethiopia	77.5	83.8	6.3
12	Ghana	35.7	63.7	28.0
13	Guinea	49.9	63.6	13.7
14	Kenya	70.5	59.9	-10.6
15	Lesotho	56.7	62.0	5.3
16	Liberia	50.8	72.3	21.5
17	Madagascar	38.8	72.8	34.0
18	Malawi	69.9	79.4	9.5
19	Mali	52.0	77.2	25.2
20	Mozambique	82.7	76.6	-6.1
21	Namibia	86.4	73.7	-12.7
22	Niger	93.3	85.3	-8.0
23	Nigeria	37.1	54.3	17.2
24	Rwanda	69.0	91.3	22.3
25	Senegal	59.1	86.5	27.4
26	Sierra Leone	50.4	68.4	18.0
27	South Africa	83.6	80.4	3.2
28	Tanzania	72.9	60.8	-12.1
29	Togo	41.7	52.9	11.2
30	Uganda	82.7	58.5	-24.2
31	Zambia	56.1	81.6	25.5
32	Zimbabwe	88.9	73.0	-15.9

Table 2.
Percentage of women currently using modern contraceptive methods who received their most recent supply or information from a public source, DHS surveys [66].

could be due to marital problems such as disapproval by the spouse or economic such as cost or health system factors such as lack of accessibility or availability to continue with the current method. Studies have shown that fear of side effects especially those associated with hormonal contraception has been reported to act as strong barriers [69–72], while other studies revealed fear of infertility, menstrual irregularities, cancer, weight gain [73–76] and spousal communication [77–79] as barriers to use contraceptives.

Sub-Saharan Africa has the highest overall discontinuation rates due to all reasons, ranging from 19.1% in Namibia to 65.5% in Guinea [66]. In this analysis, five out of twelve countries have experienced an increase in discontinuation rates. All except Nigeria with a rate of 13% had these rates less than 5%. Senegal recorded massive decline in discontinuation rate or negative 15.9% (or −15.9%) (**Figure 3**). However, at a global level, the lowest discontinuation is recorded in Papua New Guinea with a rate of rate 15.6% [80].

Concerning method switch, the same twelve countries were involved due to a variety of reasons enumerated above. Four countries recorded increases in the rates of switching, while the remaining experienced declines of up to 6.3% (or −6.3%) (**Table 3**). Rate of discontinuation due to desire to become pregnant declined in three countries, while Nigeria and Republic of Benin recorded the largest increases of up to 4.5% each (**Table 4**).

Discontinuation due to side effects declined in four countries but increased in the remaining eight (**Table 5**). The largest increase was recorded in Nigeria, 5.1%. Discontinuation due to health-related factors could be an indicator of quality of family planning services.

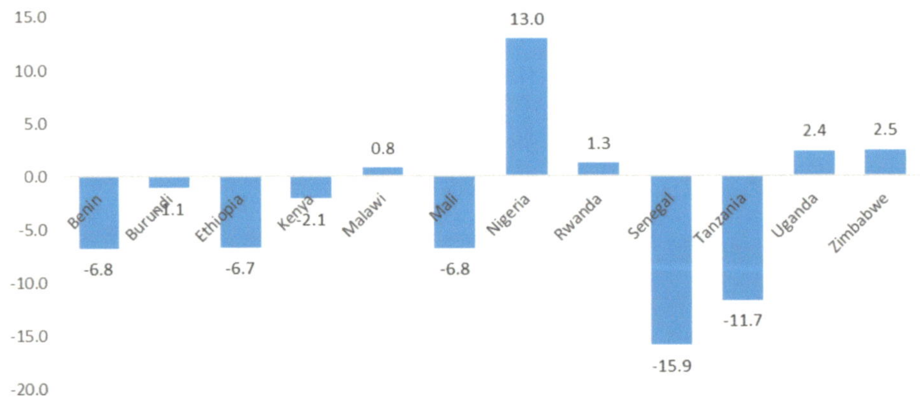

Figure 3.
Change in the first-year contraceptive discontinuation rate due to all reasons, DHS surveys.

Country	Recent	Earliest	Change
Benin	2.5	1.5	1.0
Burundi	4.6	8.1	−3.5
Ethiopia	5.8	12.1	−6.3
Kenya	10.5	7.0	3.5
Malawi	5.3	3.7	1.6
Mali	1.9	3.4	−1.5
Nigeria	4.5	4.8	−0.3
Rwanda	10.3	10.4	−0.1
Senegal	4.2	5.2	−1.0
Tanzania	6.4	9.4	−3.0
Uganda	5.0	5.2	−0.2
Zimbabwe	6.7	4.2	2.5

Table 3.
Percentage of women currently using modern contraceptive methods who discontinued by switching to another method, DHS surveys.

	Country	Earliest	Recent	Change
1	Benin	7.7	12.2	4.5
2	Burundi	9.0	9.2	0.2
3	Ethiopia	10.3	10.8	0.5
4	Kenya	4.6	4.7	0.1
5	Malawi	8.4	6.7	−1.7
6	Mali	13.8	14.8	1.0
7	Nigeria	8.2	12.7	4.5
8	Rwanda	2.7	3.9	1.2
9	Senegal	7.3	6.3	−1.0
10	Tanzania	8.4	5.1	−3.3
11	Uganda	7.5	8.8	1.3
12	Zimbabwe	4.8	5.1	0.3

Table 4.
Percentage of women currently using modern contraceptive methods who discontinued due to desire to become pregnant, DHS surveys.

	Country	Earliest	Recent	Change
1	Benin	5.9	5.8	−0.1
2	Burundi	10.6	15.2	4.6
3	Ethiopia	14.5	7.4	−7.1
4	Kenya	8.5	10.5	2.0
5	Malawi	10.5	10.6	0.1
6	Mali	10.3	10.5	0.2
7	Nigeria	2.1	7.2	5.1
8	Rwanda	10.7	10.8	0.1
9	Senegal	14.2	11.3	−2.9
10	Tanzania	11.6	9.8	−1.8
11	Uganda	15.8	18.1	2.3
12	Zimbabwe	3.6	6.0	2.4

Table 5.
Percentage of women currently using modern contraceptive methods who discontinued due to side effects, DHS surveys.

6. Factors associated with the use of modern contraception

The current body of knowledge is replete with literature on the factors associated with the use of modern contraception. Systematically, these factors are grouped into two broad categories:

1. Individual factors

2. Contextual factors

6.1 Individual factors

Education of the woman appeared as a strong and consistent predictor of contraceptive uptake. Across many studies, women with higher level of education reported current use of modern contraception compared to those with none or lower level [81–84]. Educated women are more likely to use modern contraception because it facilitates several pathways to use contraception. For instance, educated women are more likely to know where to access contraception and also more likely to be financially empowered to purchase if the need warrants. By giving her the financial and decision-making autonomy, education gives the woman the confidence to engage her spouse (husband) on discussing the need to use contraception for social, fertility and medical reasons. Age of the woman has also been found to play an important role in modern use of contraception. Younger women were found to be using less of contraception particularly if they had had no living children [79]. It is the desire of every woman to bear a child immediately after getting married most especially in high-fertility countries. After achieving the desired number of children, the use of contraception increases [85, 86]. Women who perceived their husband's disapproval of contraception are unlikely to use it partly due to cultural dominance of the husband as the sole decision-maker [72, 87]. Male partner involvement has been shown by numerous studies to positively increase use of contraception by women [88]. Also, positive male attitudes toward family planning have been reported to influence the use of contraception both from cross-sectional questionnaire and focus group discussion studies [89, 90]. Other individual-level characteristics reported to influence use of modern contraception include being employed [81, 84], religion [91–93] and spousal communication [72, 92].

6.2 Contextual factors

Broadly, the contextual factors considered here include socio-cultural, economic and health systems, specifically, place of residence, household economic status, social networks, accessible health facilities and/or health care workers providing contraception.

Women residing in urban areas have an advantage through both improved access to variety of contraception and being exposed to information channels that could positively influence utilization [92]. This urban advantage is also linked to average higher educational level of the women in urban areas as well as accessibility and being aware of facilities (both public and private) providing family planning services dotting the urban areas [71, 94, 95]. Household wealth level has also been reported to positively influence uptake of contraception. With higher household economic status, women are most likely to overcome cost-related barriers to the commodity and hidden cost of transportation and opportunity cost to obtain contraception [83]. Strong social networks among men that encourage and support use of modern contraception are a significant factor in increased use among the wives of these social networks [82, 96]. Other contextual factors known to positively increase contraceptive uptake include available and accessible facilities providing family planning services [70, 92, 97], visit by a health care worker or having a discussion with health care worker on contraception [98], cultural norms concerning fertility and contraception [92, 99, 100].

7. Conclusion

Understanding the factors beyond the individual and household characteristics that affect utilization and household characteristics that affect utilization of these important maternal health services can assist in designing the strategies and developing policies and interventions toward improvement of service utilization across SSA. This will decrease the unacceptably high maternal mortality. The determinants of reproductive health and FP services in Africa are multi-sectional and thus will require multi-sectoral approach in addressing them. Socio-cultural, health, transportation, education, empowerment and other factors will need to be on board as part of sustainable long-term approach to improve access to services and utilization. Linking poor, rural women, improving service quality and access to ANC, delivery and PNC including FP services can go a long way in increasing utilization that could further improve health outcomes and achieve SDGs.

Conflict of interest

The authors declare no conflict of interest.

Author details

Alhaji A. Aliyu* and Tukur Dahiru
Department of Community Medicine, Faculty of Clinical Sciences, College of Medical Sciences, Ahmadu Bello University, Zaria, Nigeria

*Address all correspondence to: alhajimph@gmail.com

References

[1] Solar O, Irwin A. A Conceptual Framework for Action on the Social Determinants of Health. Social Determinants of Health Discussion Paper 2. Geneva: WHO; 2010. Available from: http://www.popline.org/node/216706 [Accessed: 15 October 2019]

[2] WHO: Maternal Mortality in 2000: Estimates Developed by WHO, UNICEF and UNFPA. Geneva: World Health Organization; 2004

[3] Islam M. The safe motherhood interactive and beyond: (Editorials). Bulletin of the World Health Organization. 2007;**85**:10

[4] Pruel A, Toure A, Huguet D, Laurent Y. The quality of risk factor screening during antenatal consultation in Niger. Health Policy and Planning. 2000;**15**(1):11-16

[5] WHO. WHO Recommended Interventions for Improving Maternal and Newborn Health. Geneva: WHO; 2009

[6] Omo-Aghoja L. Sexual and reproductive health: Concepts and current status among Nigerians. African Journal of Medical and Health Sciences. 2013;**12**:103-113

[7] Horton R. Reviving reproductive health. Lancet. 2006;**368**(1549): 1595-1607

[8] WHO. WHO Recommendations on Antenatal Care for a Positive Pregnancy Experience. Geneva: WHO; 2016. Available from: http://www.who.int/iristream/10665 [Accessed: 16 July 2018]

[9] Testa J, Ouedraogo C, Prual A, Bernish D, Kone B. Determinants of risk factors associated with severe maternal morbidity: Application during antenatal consultations. Journal de Gynecologie, Obstetrique et Biologie de la Reproduction. 2002;**31**:44-50

[10] Ransjo-Arvidson AB, Chintu K, N'gandu N, Erikson B, Susu D, Christensson K, et al. Maternal and infant health problems after normal childbirth: A randomized controlled study in Zambia. Journal of Epidemiology and Community Health. 1998;**52**:385-391

[11] AbouZahr C, Berer M. When pregnancy is over: Preventing postpartum deaths and morbidity-safe motherhood initiatives: Critical issues. In: Berer M, Ravindran TKS, editors. Reproductive Health Matter. London: Great Britain-Spider Web; 1999

[12] Magadi MA, Zulu E, Brocherhoff M. The inequality of maternal health in urban sub-Saharan Africa in the 1990s. Population Studies. 2003;**57**:347-366

[13] WHO/UNICEF/UNFPA. Maternal mortality in 2000. Estimates developed by WHO, UNICEF, UNFPA. 2004

[14] Tawiah EO. Maternal health care in five sub-Saharan African countries. African Population Studies. 2011;**25**(1):1-25

[15] Tawiah EO. Determinants maternal health care in Ghana. Ghana Medical Journal. 1998;**32a**:917-925

[16] Magadi MA, Diamond I, Madise N, Smith P. Pathways of the determinants of unfavourable birth outcomes in Kenya. Journal of Biosocial Science. 2004;**36**:153-176

[17] Ram F, Singh A. Is antenatal care effective in improving maternal health in rural Uttar Pradesh? Evidence from a district level household survey. Journal of Biosocial Science. 2006;**38**:433-448

[18] Ikeako I, Onah HE, Iloabachie GC. Influence of formal education on the use of maternity services in Enugu Nigeria. Journal of Obstetrics and Gynaecology. 2006;**1**:30-34

[19] Addai I. Determinants of use of maternal-child health services in rural Ghana. Journ of Biosocial Science. 2000;**32**(1):1-15

[20] Nwakoby BN. Use of obstetric services in rural Nigeria. Journal of the Royal Society of Health. 1994;**114**:132-136

[21] Say L, Raine R. A systematic review of inequalities in the use of maternal health care in developing countries: Examining the scale of the problem and the importance of context. Bulletin of the World Health Organization. 2007;**85**:812-819

[22] McCray M. An issue of culture: The effects of daily activities on parental care utilization patterns in rural south Africa. Social Science and Medicine. 2004;**59**:1843-1855

[23] Ayanore MA, Pavlova M, Groot W. Unmet reproductive health needs among women in some West African Countries: A systematic review of outcome measures and determinants. Reproductive Health. 2016;**13**:5

[24] Leke RJI. Family Planning in Africa South of the Sahara. Available from: https://www.gfmer.ch/Books/Reproductive_Health2016:13.5

[25] Caldwell JC. Population policy: A survey of Commonwealth Africa. In: Caldwell JC, Okonjo C, editors. The Population of Tropical Africa. New York: Columbia University Press; 1968. p. 372

[26] Mario D, Basevi V, Spettoli D. What is the Effectiveness of Antenatal Care? (Supplement). Copenhagen: WHO Regional Office for Europe (Health Evidence Network Report); 2005

[27] Dansou J, Adekunle AO, Arowojolu AO. Factors associated with antenatal care services utilization patterns amongst reproductive age women in Benin Republic: An analysis of 2011-12 Benin Republic's DHS data. The Nigerian Postgraduate Medical Journal. 2017;**24**:67-74

[28] Damstadt GL, Bhutta ZA, Cousens S, Adam T, Walker N, de Bernis L. Lancet Neonatal Steering Team. Evidenced-based cost effective interventions: How many newborn babies can we save? Lancet. 2005;**365**:977-978

[29] Wang W, Alva S, Wang S, Fort A. Levels and Trends in the Use of Maternal Health Services in Developing Countries. ICF Macro: Calver ton, MD, USA; 2011

[30] Mpembeni R, Kilewo J, Leshabari M, Siriel N, Massawe S, Jahn A, et al. Use pattern of maternal health services and determinants of skilled care during delivery in Southern Tanzania: Implications for achievement of MDG-5 targets. BMC Pregnancy and Childbirth. 2007;**7**:29

[31] Fotso JC, Even A, Oronje R. Provision and use of maternal health services among urban poor women in Kenya: What do we know and what can we do? Journal of Urban Health. 2008;**85**(3):428-442

[32] Obago IT. The Role of Antenatal Care in Predicting Health Facility Delivery Among Women in Kenya: Further Analysis of Data from the 2008-09 KDHS. DHS Working Papers No. 86. Calverton, Maryland, USA: ICF International; 2013

[33] Ochako R, Fotso JC, Ikamari L, Khasakhala A. Utilization of maternal health services among young women in Kenya: Insights from Kenya demographic health survey 2003. BMC Pregnancy and Childbirth. 2011;**11**:1

[34] Babalola S, Fatusi A. Determinants of use of maternal health service in Nigeria-Looking beyond individual and household factors. BMC Pregnancy and Childbirth. 2009;**9**:43

[35] Simkhada B, Van Teijlingren ER, Porter M, Simkhada P. Factors affecting the utilization of antenatal care in developing countries: Systematic review of the literature. Journal of Advanced Nursing. 2007;**63**(3):244-260

[36] Kabir M, Iliyasu Z, Abubakar IS, Sani A. Determinants of utilization of antenatal care services in Kumbotso village, Northern Nigeria. Tropical Doctor. 2005;**35**:110-111

[37] Adamu YM, Salihu HM. Barriers to the use of antenatal and obstetric care services in rural Kano, Nigeria. Journal of Obstetrics and Gynaecology. 2002;**22**(6):600-603

[38] Mekonnen Y, Mekonnen A. Factors influencing the use of maternal health care services in Ethiopia. Journal of Health, Population and Nutrition. 2003;**21**(4):374-382

[39] Mathole T, Lindmark G, Majoko F, Ahlberg BM. A qualitative study of women's perspectives of antenatal care in rural area of Zimbabwe. Midwifery. 2004;**20**(2):122-132

[40] Ganle JK, Obang B, Segbetia AY, Mwinyuri V, Yeboah JY, Baatiema L. How intra familial decision-making affects women's access to, and use of maternal health care services in Ghana: A qualitative study. BMC Pregnancy and Childbirth. 2015;**15**:173

[41] WHO. The World Health Report 2005-Make Every Mother and Child Care Count. WHO; 2005

[42] WHO Skilled Attendant at Birth-2006 Updates. Geneva: WHO; 2006. Available from: http://www.who.int/reproductive-health/global-monitoring/skilled-attendant [Accessed: 28 October 2019]

[43] Abouzhar C. Maternal mortality overview. In: Murray CJ, Lopez AD, editors. Health Dimensions, Sex and Reproduction. Geneva: WHO; 1998. pp. 111-164

[44] Gabrysch S, Campbell OMR. Still too far to walk: Literature review of the determinants of delivery service use. BMC Pregnancy and Childbirth. 2009;**9**:34

[45] Lawn JE, Cousens S, Zupan J. 4 million neonatal deaths: When? Where? Why? Lancet. 2005;**365**(9462):891-900

[46] National Population Commission (NPC) Nigeria and ICF. Nigeria Demographic and Rockville, Maryland USA: NPC and ICF; 2019

[47] Zimbabwe National Statistics Agency and ICF. Zimbabwe Demographic and Health Survey 2015 Final Report. Rockville, Maryland, USA: Zimbabwe National Statistics Agency (ZIMSTA) and ICF International. 2016

[48] Ghana Statistical Service (GSS), Ghana Health Service (GHS) and ICF. Ghana Maternal Health Service, 2017. Accra, Ghana: GSS, GHS and ICF; 2018

[49] Ministry of Health, Community Development, Gender, Elderly and Children (MOHCDGEC) [Tanzania Mainland], Ministry of Health (MOH) [Zanzibar], National Bureau of Statistics (NBS), Office of the Chief Government Statistician (OCGS) and ICF. Tanzania Demographic and Health Survey and Malaria Indicator Survey (TDHS-MIS) 2015-16. Dares Salaam and Rockville, Maryland, USA: MOHCDGEC, MoH, NBS, OCGS and ICF; 2016

[50] Tarekegn SM, Lieberman LS, Gredraitis V. Determinants of maternal health service utilization in Ethiopia:

Analysis of the 2011 Ethiopian Demographic and health Survey. BMC Pregnancy and Childbirth. 2014;**14**:161

[51] Aliyu AA. Family planning services in Africa: The successes and challenges. In: Amarin ZO, editor. Family Planning. London, UK: IntechOpen; 2018

[52] Burgard S. Race and pregnancy-related care in Brazil and South Africa. Social Science and Medicine. 2004;**59**:1123

[53] CSF (Ethiopia) and ICF International: Ethiopia Demographic and Health Survey 2011. Addis Ababa, Ethiopia and Calverton, Maryland, USA: Central Statistical Agency and ICF International; 2012

[54] Mwangi W, Gachuno O, Desai M, Obor D, Were V, Odhiambo F, et al. Uptake take of skill dance along the continuous of care in rural Western Kenya: Selected analysis from Global Health Initiative Survey 2012. Pregnancy and Childbirth. 2018;**18**:175

[55] Shiferaw S, Spigt M, Godefroij M, Mel Kanu Y, Tekie M. Why do women prefer home births in Ethiopia? BMC Pregnancy and Child Birth. 2013;**13**:5

[56] Gaje AJ. Barriers to the utilization of maternal health care in rural Mali. Social Science and Medicine. 2007;**65**:1666-1682

[57] Gabysch S, Cox CS, Campbell OMR. The influence of distance and level of care on delivery place in rural Zambia: A study of linked national data in a geographic information system. PLoS Medicine. 2011;**8**(1):1-12

[58] Hodgkin D. Household characteristics affecting where mothers deliver in rural Kenya. Health Economics. 1996;**5**(4):333-340

[59] Abuozahr C, Wardlaw T. Maternal mortality at the end of a decade: Signs of progress? Bulletin of the World Health Organization. 2001;**79**:561-568

[60] WHO, editor. Postpartum Care of the Mothers and Newborn: A Practical Guide. Volth ed. Geneva: WHO; 1958. WHO/RHT/MSM/983

[61] WHO. WHO Recommendations on Postnatal Care of Mothers and Newborn. Geneva: WHO; 2013

[62] Rwabufigiri BN, Mukamurigo J, Thomson DR, Hedt-Gautier BL, Semasaka JP. Factors associated with postnatal care utilization in Rwanda: A secondary analysis of 2010 Demographic and Health Survey Data. BMC Pregnancy and Childbirth. 2016;**16**:122

[63] National Bureau of Statistics of Tanzania ICF International. Tanzania Demographic and Health Survey 2010. Available from: http://dhsprogram/pubs/pdf/FR243 [Accessed: 25 November 2019]

[64] Aminah K. Factors Determining the Utilization of Postpartum Care Services in Uganda, Ugandan Demographic and Health Survey (UDHS). 2006

[65] Ahmed S, Creanga AA, Gilespie DG, Tsui AO. Economic status, education and empowerment: Implications for maternal health service utilization in developing countries. PLoS One. 2010;**5**(6):e11190

[66] Demographic and Health Survey (DHS) Reports. Available from: https://dhsprogram.com/publications/index.ctm

[67] Khan S, Mishra V, Arnold F, Abderrahim N. Contraceptive Trends in Developing Countries. DHS Comparative Reports No. 16. Macro International Inc: Calverton, Maryland, USA; 2007

[68] Gareme M. Family planning and fertility decline in Africa: From 1950-2010. In: Amarin Z, editor. Family Planning. Rijeka: IntechOpen; 2018

[69] Abiodun OM, Balogun OR. Sexual activity and contraceptive use among young female students of tertiary educational institutions in Ilorin, Nigeria. Contraception. 2009;**79**(2):146-149

[70] Teye JK. Modern contraceptive use among women in the Asuogyaman district of Ghana: Is reliability more important than health concerns? African Journal of Reproductive Health. 2013;**17**(2):58-71

[71] Asekun-Olarinmoye E, Adebimbe W, Bamidele J, Odu O, Asekum-Olarinmoye I, Ojofeitimi E. Barriers to use of modern contraceptives among women in an inner city area of Oshogbo metropolis, Osun State, Nigeria. International Journal of Women's Health. 2013;**5**:647-655

[72] Nwachukwu I, Obasi OO. Use of modern birth control methods among rural communities in Imo State, Nigeria. African Journal of Reproductive Health. 2008;**12**(1):101-108

[73] Ugboaja JO. Contraceptive choices and practices among urban women in south eastern Nigeria. Nigerian Journal of Medicine. 2011;**20**(3):360-365

[74] Ikeme ACC, Ezegwui HU, Uzodimma AC. Knowledge, attitude and use of emergency contraception among female undergraduates in Eastern Nigeria. Journal of Obstetrics and Gynaecology. 2005;**25**(5):491-493

[75] Chipeta EK, Chimwaza W, Kalilani-Phiri L. Contraceptive knowledge, beliefs and attitudes in rural Malawi: Misinformation, misbeliefs and misconceptions. Malawi Medical Journal. 2010;**22**(2):38-41

[76] Haddad LB, Cwiak C, Jamieson JD, Feldacker C, Tweya H, Hosseinipour M, et al. Contraceptive adherence among HIV-infected women in Malawi: A randomized controlled trial of the copper intrauterine device and depot medroxyprogesterone acetate. Contraception. 2013;**88**(6):737-743

[77] Iklaki CU, Ekubua JE, Abasiattai A, Massey EA, Itam IH. Spousal communication in contraceptive decisions among antenatal patients in Calabar, south eastern Nigeria. Nigerian Journal of Medicine. 2005;**14**(4): 405-407

[78] Omideyi AK, Akinyemi AI, Aina OI, Adeyemi AB, Fadeyibi OA, Bamiwuye SO. Contraceptive practice, unwanted pregnancies and induced abortion in Southwest Nigeria. Global Public Health. 2011;**6**(Suppl 1):S52-S72

[79] Bulto G, Zewdie T, Beyen T. Demand for long acting and permanent contraceptive methods and associated factors among married women of reproductive age group in Debre Markos Town, North West Ethiopia. BMC Women's Health. 2014;**14**(1):46

[80] National Statistical Office (NSO) [Papua New Guinea] and ICP. Papua New Guinea Demographic and Health Survey 2016-18. Port Moresby, Papua New Guinea and Rockville, Maryland, USA: NSO and ICF; 2019

[81] Palamuleni ME. Socio-economic and demographic factors affecting contraceptive use in Malawi. African Journal of Reproductive Health. 2013;**17**(3):91-104

[82] Paz-Soldan VA. How family planning ideas are spread within social groups in rural Malawi. Studies in Family Planning. 2004;**35**(4):275-290

[83] Crissman HP, Adanu RM, Harlow SD. Women's sexual empowerment and contraceptive use

in Ghana. Studies in Family Planning. 2012;**43**(3):201-212

[84] Ijadunola MY. Male involvement in family planning decision making in Ile-Ife, Osun State, Nigeria. African Journal of Reproductive Health. 2010;**14**(4):43-50

[85] Avidime S, Aku-Akai L, Mohammed AZ, Adaji S, Shittu OO, Ejembi CL. Fertility intentions, contraceptive awareness and contraceptive use among women in three communities of Northern Nigeria. African Journal of Reproductive Health. 2010;**14**(3):65-70

[86] Peer N, Morojele N, London L. Factors associated with contraceptive use in a rural area in Western Cape Province. South African Medical Journal. 2013;**103**(6):406

[87] Orji EO, Ojofeitimi EO, Olanrewaju BA. The role of men in family planning decision-making in rural and urban Nigeria. The European Journal of Contraception & Reproductive Health Care. 2007;**12**(1):70-75

[88] Ajah LO. Male partner involvement in female contraceptive choices in Nigeria. Journal of Obstetrics and Gynaecology: The Journal of the Institute of Obstetrics and Gynaecology. 2015;**35**:628-631

[89] Bukar M, Audu BM, Usman HA, El-Nafaty AU, Massa AA, Melah GS. Gender attitude to the empowerment of women: An independent right to contraceptive acceptance, choice and practice. Journal of Obstetrics and Gynaecology. 2013;**33**(2):180-183

[90] Izugbara C, Ibisomi L, Ezeh AC, Mandara M. Gendered interests and poor spousal contraceptive communication in Islamic northern Nigeria. The Journal of Family Planning and Reproductive Health Care. 2010;**36**(4):219-224

[91] Doctor HV, Phillips JF, Sakeah E. The influence of changes in women's religious affiliation on contraceptive use and fertility among the Kassena-Nankana of northern Ghana. Studies in Family Planning. 2009;**40**(2):113-122

[92] Audu BM, El-Nafaty AU, Bako AG, Melah GS, Mairiga AG, Kullima AA. Attitude of Nigerian women to contraceptive use by men. Journal of Obstetrics and Gynaecology. 2008;**28**(6):621-625

[93] Keele JJ, Forste R, Flake DF. Hearing native voices: Contraceptive use in Matenwe Village, East Africa. African Journal of Reproductive Health. 2005;**9**(1):32-41

[94] Polisi A, Grebrehanna E, Tesfaye G, Asefa F. Modern contraceptive utilization among female ART attendees in health facility of Gimbie town, West Ethiopia. Reproductive Health. 2014;**11**(1):30

[95] Prata N, Weidert K, Sreenivas A. Meeting the need: Youth and family planning in sub-Saharan Africa. Contraception. 2013;**88**(1):83-90

[96] Chimbiri AM. The condom is an 'intruder' in marriage: Evidence from rural Malawi. Social Science and Medicine. 2007;**64**(5):1102-1115

[97] Marrone G, Abdul-Rahman L, De Connick Z, Johansson A. Predictors of contraceptive use among female adolescents in Ghana. African Journal of Reproductive Health. 2014;**18**(1):102-109

[98] Kabagenyi A, Jennings L, Reid A. Barriers to male involvement in contraceptive uptake and reproductive health services: A qualitative study of men and women's perceptions in two rural districts in Uganda. Reproductive Health. 2014;**11**:1-10

[99] Anguzu R, Tweheyo R, Sekandi JN, Zalwango V, Muhumuza C, Tusiima S, et al. Knowledge and attitudes towards use of long acting reversible contraceptives among women of reproductive age in Lubaga division, Kampala district, Uganda. BMC Research Notes. 2014;7:153

[100] Ejembi CL, Dahiru T, Aliyu AA. Contextual Factors Influencing Modern Contraceptive Use in Nigeria. DHS Working Papers No. 120. Rockville, Maryland, USA: ICF International; 2015

Chapter 4

Planning Methods in Ecuador's Indigenous People

Yaroslava Robles-Bykbaev, Nina Naula, Javier Cornejo-Reyes, Ana Parra, Vladimir Robles-Bykbaev, Blas Garzón and Jorge Galán

Abstract

Sexual and reproductive health (SRH) is a fundamental human right that implies knowledge and exercise of sexual and reproductive rights (SSR). Among the latter are access to knowledge and use of contraceptive methods; therefore, SSR should be experienced as a constant experience that allows women to achieve full satisfaction and security in their sexual and reproductive sphere through their subjectivity, their body, and their social and cultural life. Knowing about family planning allows having the desired number of children determining the interval between pregnancies and choosing the contraceptive method according to the social, cultural and psychological beliefs, needs and conditions of each woman. However, indigenous women from Canton Cañar (Ecuador) have less access and knowledge to contraceptive methods, mainly due to the influence of social, cultural, religious and economic factors, among others. The lack of information about family planning in indigenous populations of the South of Ecuador has motivated this study; through a medical-anthropological approach, it is intended to determine what is the preference regarding contraceptive methods in indigenous Cañari women in the context of the Cañari culture and what are their perceptions regarding such methods.

Keywords: planning methods, indigenous peoples, Cañari population, indigenous women, Ecuador

1. Introduction

Health is a fundamental human right, SRH is a part of health, and this gives the reason for SRR to also be a fundamental human right [1]. The term "reproductive rights" was made public at the First International Conference on Women's Health carried out in Amsterdam, Holland, in 1984 [2], whereas the term "sexual rights" was introduced as a negotiation strategy at the International Conference on Population and Development (ICPD) in 1994, with the purpose of guaranteeing the inclusion of reproductive rights in the final version of the El Cairo Declaration and Action Program [2]. In 1997, the World Declaration of Sexual Rights was formulated at the World Congress of Sexology (Valencia-Spain). It was later ratified at the General Convention of the Sexology Association (WAS) during the XV Sexology Congress carried out in Paris.

The Organización Mundial de la Salud (OMS) [3] declared that sexual health is a state of physical, mental and social welfare related to sexuality. It demands a positive and careful treatment of sexuality and sexual relations, as well as the possibility of having pleasant and safe experiences that are free from coercion, discrimination and violence. The OMS precept on sexual health is exclusive, biased and oriented toward the western paradigm, since it does not correspond to the local reality of the Original Peoples of Ecuador such as the Cañari, determined by bio-psycho-socio-cultural factors and economics such as ethnicity (especially indigenous and mestizo), religion (Catholic, Christian, Evangelical and charismatic groups, among others), literacy, social class, level of education, work activity and profession, among others. The aforementioned factors determine the way and lifestyle of the indigenous women of Cañar, their perception of SRH and the cultural imagery through which social construction on the use of contraceptive methods takes place.

The ways and lifestyles of Cañari women have a direct "relationship with the land and fertility, as well as with physical spaces considered feminine," since they are assigned for physical and social reproduction in the community [4]. This task of reproduction prevents access to free-form contraceptive methods if they are single [5] or adolescents (18 years), since they are frowned upon by the community and are stigmatized. Therefore, the religious and cultural precepts of the Cañaris communities are focused on control [6] regarding the exercise of their SRR.

Cañari indigenous adolescents and young adult women have greater difficulties in accessing knowledge and care in contraception due to the taboo issue that SRH represents, but also due to traditional paradigms on the role of sexual reproduction, since in indigenous communities of the Ecuador the idea that sexuality is reserved for reproduction still prevails, and the generational continuities crossed by the power relations of the gender system are reinforced [7–9]. Specifically, because the house is considered a sacred and immutable group of male ancestry that controls access and management of symbolic reproduction related to fertility [10], and subordinates the symbolic representation of women towards the Nature, therefore, is a generator of life and a naturally reproductive subject [11].

Within the value system of the Cañari culture, the generational hierarchy within the female gender plays a fundamental role, since respect from one generation to another forbids the dialog between mothers and daughters about the use of contraceptive methods, due to a generational role assigned to women according to their life cycle. Therefore, it is forbidden to talk about sexuality and birth control methods ("take care" in terms of the indigenous community of Cañar) among older adult women, and young adults and adolescents.

Not being able to talk freely between women of one generation (adolescents and young adults) and those of another generation (mature adults and older adults) may be related to modesty as an acetic value within the value system of the Cañari culture governed by the influence of religion. Indeed, modesty is related to a form of social control mainly for the censorship of what is related to sexuality, therefore chastity, and also for its erotic connotation [12–14]. In other words, modesty plays a role as a sobering element for the redirection of indigenous sexual behavior, since it allows values such as dignity and honor to be achieved [15].

Shyness as a social value allows to build and achieve a stereotype of biological and social woman; therefore, it is through the body of indigenous women that the experience of social control of modesty or embodiment[1] is manifested, so that this body is the existential basis so that said social control can be generated and

[1] It consists of living, with and through the human body, a set of emotions and sensations we experiment throughout our lives [16].

reproduced collectively through the intersubjective experiences [17] of the Cañari culture. In the case of the indigenous women of Cañar, modesty in relation to body management has its essence in the tendency to hide sexual values so as not to turn the body into an object of pleasure [18] without permission and theocratic recognition of religion, for example, Catholic, Christian and Evangelical, among others, through consecrated union in the church (ecclesiastical marriage).

Body shame or embarrassment arises as a result of the body, since it occurs in relation to some aspect of the body or body management [19]; specifically, the female body continues to be a place of shame for women; it is associated with passions and uncontrolled appetites and with something dirty and polluting [20]. That is, it constitutes the social, biological and cultural site where the intersubjectivities of mature and older women, families, men and subjects of the indigenous Cañari society discipline it, and thus socially control the behavior of adolescent and young adult women, as well as single, divorced or separated women to prevent them from experiencing sexuality related to family planning. Since the female body that has not been sacralized through ecclesiastical marriage, and by the mere fact of being a female body, becomes an impure space.

Currently, the society of the Cañari culture still exercises social and biological control in the body of the indigenous women of Cañar, that is why Cañari society can accept birth control for women, as a normative and socially accepted behavior, only if women are married. This phenomenon already took place in Quito, Ecuador, in 1970 [21], since the main group of attention for family planning was women who already had children, most of them married, which reaffirmed the exercise of sexuality only under the conjugal mandate. According to the Organización Panamericana de la Salud (OPS) and the Comisión Económica para América Latina y el Caribe (CEPAL), in Ecuador, between 67% and 90% of indigenous youth reside mostly in rural areas, and they also have social exclusion, determined by schooling (4–6 years of study approved) [22]. Being a young indigenous woman and residing in a rural sector together with having an early active sexual life will become indicators of risk for SRH, exclusion, poverty and difficulty for living conditions.

The start of an active sexual life of teenagers at an early age implies risks such as unwanted pregnancy, sexually transmitted infections, clandestine abortions and social segregation, among other problems. It is estimated that in Latin America 50% of young people under 17 are sexually active [22]. In fact, in Ecuador, teenagers' sexual relations start at the age of 15 [23, 24]. In the case of teenagers' fertility (15–19 years old), an alarming increase of 11% between 1999 and 2004 and between 2007 and 2012 [25] has been observed in Ecuador.

In most nonwestern countries, and especially in indigenous contexts, women reach the state of biological and social adulthood with marriage and motherhood at a stage in life that—according to western chronological criteria—could be categorized as adolescence. In this way, the right to marry is connected to biological maturity in traditional societies [22]. Despite the fact that in indigenous communities the acquired right to access family planning is instrumentalized and admitted by marriage, women do not have the same freedom to exercise their SRR, including that of family planning.

Teenage women, young adults and single mature adults who choose a family planning method are socially singled out. Well, sexuality is repressed, since sexual relations before marriage is seen as a lack of honor and a risk for women [26]. Therefore, the women's body is relate to something dirty and polluting, for that reason that mentioned body plays again a fundamental role as a social and biological space for socialization of the experience of cultural values. In other words, the passions and and uncontrolled appetites that those women can have must be social controlled by the Cañari culture. Even more so, if they are single indigenous women, they are socially stigmatized or singled out; in fact, according to the

Ministerio de Salud Pública del Ecuador (MSP), this social phenomenon stands out, since single mothers are the target of aggression and contempt in the community; and girls are physically and psychologically punished and are often expelled from home and from the community [27].

For their part, married indigenous women who have children can opt for family planning; in addition, society assigns the role of motherhood as a central component of their existence and socially grants them prestige and social recognition [27]. We will then say that the prevailing cultural system, the model of social control based on religious asceticism, the generational hierarchy in the female gender, patriarchal domination and belonging to the indigenous ethnic group in localities of Cañar influence access to knowledge and care in SRH and SSR, and therefore access to family planning methods.

According to OMS [3], it is calculated that, at world level, 214 million women of childbearing age in developing countries want to postpone or stop procreation, but they do not use any modern contraceptive method. However, in Ecuador, according to INEC [28, 29], the indigenous population has the lowest knowledge of contraceptive methods (34.7% of a total of 221.558). Regarding the prevalence of contraceptives and demand for satisfactory family planning [30], a more substantial dependence on traditional methods is observed in Ecuador in women aged 15 to 49. In the case of contraceptive methods, indigenous women prefer the use of rhythm or calendar (24.6%), ligature (23.6%), IUD/IUS (copper spiral "T") (19.1%), injection (16.4%), abstinence (6.7%), contraceptive pill (5.3%) and, finally, condom (3.9%). From their part, mestizo women prefer tubal ligation or female sterilization (35.9%), contraceptive pill (18.7%), rhythm (15%), IUD/IUS (14%), injection (9.5%), condom (4.2%) and abstinence (1.2%).

The rhythm method is currently not recommended or is proscribed as being ineffective [31]. Furthermore, the fact that indigenous women prefer such a contraceptive method is a trend that reflects less access to knowledge and family planning. The preference for tubal ligation and the preference for the rhythm method reveal the place that women occupy with regard to the subject of rights [32]; however, the strong religious influence reflects how women, indigenous people and their partners consider the use of contraceptive methods as a sin, and for their part, men consider that their partners can return to being adulterous [33].

1.1 Some data about the province and city of Cañar

In the province of Cañar (located in southern Ecuador), 15.2% of its population identifies itself as indigenous, while 76.7% identifies itself as mestizos [34]. It is a culturally representative province of Ecuador regarding customs, history and archeological remains. In the Cañar canton (located in the Cañar Province in the south of the country), there are 12 parishes: Cañar, Chontamarca, Chorocopte, Ducur, General Morales, Gualleturo, Honorato Vásquez, Ingapirca, Juncal, San Antonio, Ventura and Zhud.

According to the Municipio Intercultural del Cañar [35], this canton has around 58,185 inhabitants, and 40% of the population is indigenous, represented mainly by the Cañari ethnic group. The Cañari people speak Kichwa and Spanish. The identities of each indigenous people of the Cañari culture take place through the colonial present, but also with some influence from the pre-Inca past [36]. Furthermore, expressions, manifestations and their cultural value system are subject to resignifications due to processes of cultural syncretism.

In 2015, according to the Secretaría Nacional de Planificación y Desarrollo (SENPLADES) [37], the illiteracy rate for the indigenous population of the Cañar Province represented 42.78% and the poverty rate 95.2%. According to CEPAL [38], in 2001, the global fertility rate was 4.6 in the indigenous population in the province of Cañar, while for 2015, according to (SENPLADES), the number of teenage pregnancies (15–19 years) in Cañar [37] reached 11% in the province of Cañar.

With the exposed background about cultural phenomenology, which has allowed to partially understand how the perception of sexuality takes place and, as a part of it, how the indigenous women of Cañar manage family planning, our interest is to determine their preferences regarding contraceptive methods, considering the fact that there is scarce information about it. For this purpose, a descriptive-exploratory study was conducted (diagnosis phase) that focused on determining the perception indigenous women, aged 19–59, of the rural areas of Juncal and Ingapirca and the urban area of Cañar have about the use of and preference for contraceptive methods.

2. Methodology and design

This was a descriptive-exploratory study because information about family planning in the indigenous communities located to the South of Ecuador, such as Cañar, is scarce and insufficient, especially due to their biological position.

Data gathering was done by administering a previously validated survey through the Cronbach's alpha test (0.7). This survey was administered in the city of Cañar in 3 occasions during 3 months, considering the fact that SRH is a taboo and reaching a quotient of Cronbach's alpha higher than 0.7 was not possible. As previously stated, on the one hand, it is necessary to consider the difficulty of accessing a social construct about SRH within the system of values of this population. On the other hand, this is an exploratory study (diagnosis phase or baseline) and there is not enough information about this population's preferences regarding birth control methods, and due to the structure of their cultural system and cosmogony, access to information is restricted by the marked complexity that the cultural construct of sexuality represents. For this reason, it was decided to work with a quotient of Cronbach's alpha of 0.7.

Sampling was done randomly to 25 women who identified themselves as indigenous. It was checked that they had a level of elementary, high school and higher education. The surveys were applied in high social activity strategic zones in three parishes: Cañar (urban), Ingapirca and Juncal (rural). Additionally, accessing to the next parishes was easier (see **Table 1**), considering the fact that, in general, it is not easy to gather information in indigenous communities because local and/or foreign researchers usually get data but people disapprove of this:

- In the community of Yaculoma, which belongs to the parish of Juncal, surveys were applied to indigenous women attending the Unidad Educativa Intercultural de Juncal.
- At the cattle square and the clothes market of the urban parish of Cañar.
- At the community of Vendeleche belonging to the parish of Ingapirca.

The majority of the Cañari indigenous women interviewed belong to the parishes of Ingapirca (10) and Cañar (8) (see **Table 1**) and they speak both languages: Spanish and Kichwa.

The analysis of information was done by using "R" open software, version 1.1.456. A descriptive statistical analysis was done (measurements of central and dispersion tendency) because it was necessary to start with a diagnosis phase of the preference the indigenous women of the city of Cañar have regarding the use of contraceptives.

Parishes	Communities	Indigenous women	Total	%
Cañar	Cañar	2	8	32
	Cañaribamba	1		
	Coriurco	3		
	Quilloac	2		
Chorocopte	La Capilla	2	4	16
	Tretón	2		
El Tambo	Coyoctor	1	1	4
Gualleturo	Gasa	1	1	4
Honorato Vásquez	Sigsihuayco	1	1	4
Ingapirca	Cebadas	6	10	40
	Chuguin Grande	1		
	Cochapamba	1		
	Masanqui	1		
	Sisid	1		
		25	**25**	**100%**

Table 1.
The table shows the Cañaris parishes were the surveys have been applied to indigenous women.

Surveys were applied to volunteer indigenous women of Cañar of any marital status, aged 19–59, with a level of elementary, high school or higher education. Volunteer participants signed the informed consent before participating in this study. Surveys were applied by a previously trained team of women, and one of the team collaborators was a Kichwa native speaker and supported the rest or the team to access the communities.

3. Results

It is worth mentioning that the results obtained should be considered taking into account several variables: age, marital status, years of study, the level of education and current occupation, and also, all respondents were indigenous and Catholic.

The age range of respondents was between 19 and 59 years. It was observed that the average pregnancy per woman was 3.08, and the pregnancy range was from 0 to 8 children, 2.72 being the average. Regarding the level of education of respondents, 15 women had elementary school education, 3 women had high school instruction and 7 had a higher education degree. In relation to their marital status, 22 women were married, 1 woman had free union relationship and 2 were single.

We asked some questions in order to understand what is the preference regarding contraceptive methods in Cañari indigenous women and what are their perceptions regarding such methods:

1. How many children do Cañari indigenous women have?

2. What is the most widely identified contraceptive method by the indigenous women of Cañar, according to the community they are from, their level of education and age?

3. What family planning method is the most widely used and which age group of women prefers this method?

4. How many children do women who have generally had tubal ligation have, how old were they when they decided to have tubal ligation and what is their level of education?

5. What is the age to begin the use of contraceptives in Cañari indigenous women, and why?

It is important to mention here that the results obtained showed that the women were engaged in the following activities: farmer (28%), housewife (40%), merchants (8%), public servant (8%), teacher (8%), physiotherapy assistant (4%) and student (4%). The 80% of housewife women respondents and the 100% of the farmer women respondents have elementary school education. The Cañari indigenous women respondents above mentioned belongs to the communities of Cañar (8), Chorocopte (4), Tambo (1), Gualleturo (1), 14 Honorato Vásquez (1) and the parish of Ingapirca (10) (see **Figure 1**).

3.1 How many children do Cañari indigenous women have?

Women having a higher number of children are those who have elementary school education, especially indigenous women between 49 and 59 years old (see **Table 2**), probably due to the fact that only 193.5 (estimated number in thousands) cases of sterilized women between 15 and 49 years old were registered in Ecuador until 1987 [39]. For this reason, women living in rural areas of Ecuador in the 1990s (30 years ago) did not know much about tubal ligation as a contraceptive method. Consequently, it was not a well-known birth control option; on the other hand, it was fundamental to have large families so that children can contribute to

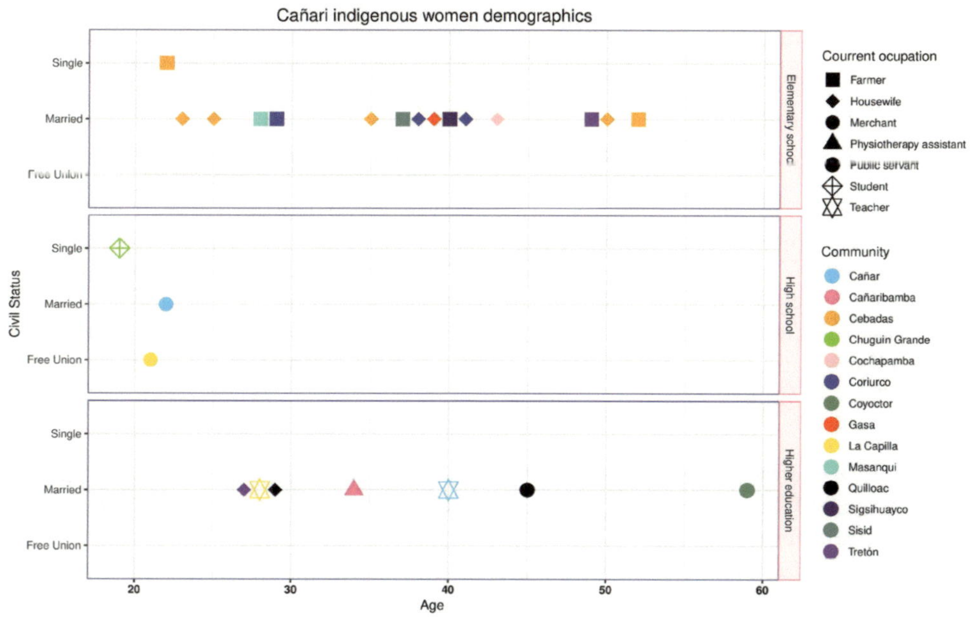

Figure 1.
The panel shows how indigenous women have been categorized according to their marital status, scholarity, current occupation and community. As ***Table 1*** *shows, most women are married and have elementary school and higher education, are from the communities of Cebadas and Coriurco, and are farmers.*

Age group	Marital status	Higher education	Elementary school	High school	Number of children
19–28	Free Union			1 (1.47%)	10 (14.71%)
	Married	2 (2.94%)	5 (7.35%)	1 (1.47%)	
	Single		1 (1.47%)		
29–38	Married	3 (4.41%)	11 (16.80%)		14 (20.59%)
39–48	Married	5 (7.35%)	21 (30.88%)		26 (38.24%)
49–59	Married	2 (2.94%)	16 (23.53%)		18 (26.47%)
		12 (16.76%)	54 (79.41%)	2 (2.94%)	68 (100.0%)

Table 2.
Number of children that indigenous women of Cañar have according to age group and education level.

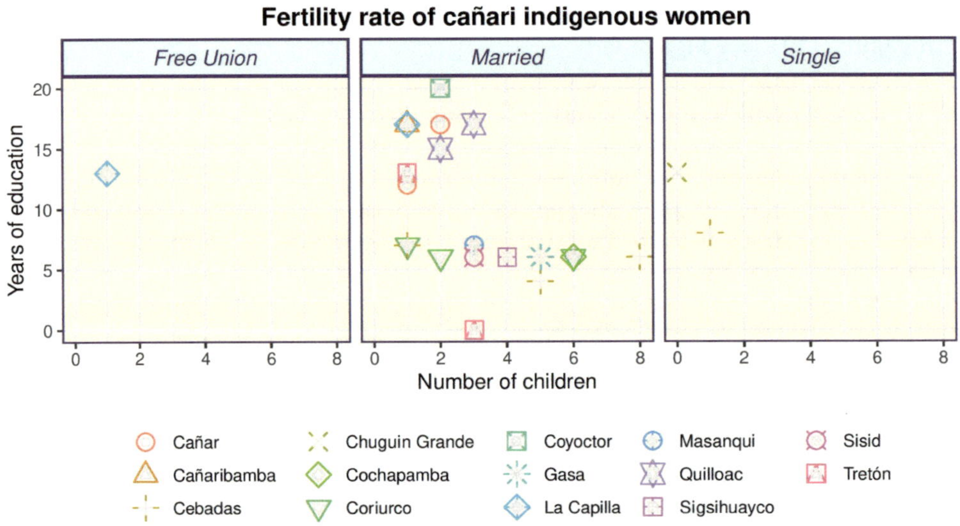

Figure 2.
Number of children that Cañari indigenous women have according to level of education and civil status.

agricultural and livestock tasks, especially in rural areas. Currently, there are still indigenous communities in Cañar, where women having a higher number of children, that is, between 5 and 8 children, are those from the rural parishes of Cebadas, Cochapamba, Coriurco and Gasa, and they have between 5 and 6 years of education (elementary school), while single women or women who have a free union relationship have 1 child and are from Chuguin Grande, Cebadas and La Capilla (see **Figure 2**).

3.2 What is the most widely identified contraceptive method by the indigenous women of Cañar, according to the community they are from, their level of education level and age?

The two most widely known contraceptive methods by the Cañari indigenous women between 19 and 59 years old are tubal ligation (24%) and hormonal injection (24%), followed by the contraceptive pill (16%) and no method (8%). It is important to say that Cebadas is the community that most identify contraceptive methods (24%) as: hormonal injection, implant and tubal ligation (see **Table 3**).

Contraceptive methods	Elementary school	High school	Higher education	Total
All			1	1
Hormonal injection	5		1	6
Various	1	2	1	4
Implant	1			1
IUD/IUS			1	1
Pill	1		3	4
Tubal ligation	6			6
None	1	1		2
	15	3	7	25

Table 3.
Contraceptive methods identified by Cañari indigenous women.

Tubal ligation, for its part, has been identified as an inexpensive method, which is easy to access, allows family planning and avoids teenage pregnancy. Cañari indigenous women also say that it is easy to access hormonal injections, which allow family planning and avoid teenage pregnancy. Regarding contraceptive pills, indigenous women know about the last two advantages indicated above. There is also the perception that not using a contraceptive method is inexpensive. Finally, pills and/or hormonal injections are considered to be inexpensive and comfortable (see **Figure 3**).

3.3 What family planning method is the most widely used and which age group of Cañari indigenous women prefers this method?

The contraceptive methods the indigenous married women of the city of Cañar who were surveyed prefer are tubal ligation (36%), none (28%), injections (12%), implants (12%), contraceptive pill (8%) and rhythm method (4%). The community where contraceptives are most widely used is Cebadas (24%) (see **Table 4**). It must be considered that most respondents were married (22–25 years old; see **Table 1**). This is worth noticing because single women did not want to participate to avoid being identified and stigmatized and criticized by the people of the community, as it was stated in the theoretical section of this discussion. It is also necessary to highlight that all the respondents declared themselves to be Catholic and, as it was

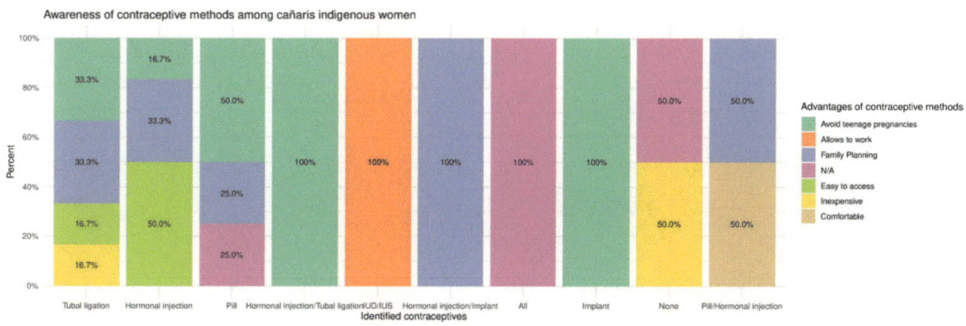

Figure 3.
Notice that the indigenous women of Cañar know about hormonal injection and/or tubal ligation, as well as implants, as valid options to avoid teenage pregnancy, IUD/IUS as a method that allows them to work, and hormonal injection and/or implants as methods that allow them to plan their pregnancies.

Contraceptive methods	Single	Free union	Married	Total
Hormonal injection			3	3
Implant	1	1	1	3
Pill			2	2
Rhythm method			1	1
Tubal ligation			9	9
None	1		6	7
	2	1	22	25

Table 4.
Contraceptive methods used by Cañari indigenous women.

stated before, they have a system of social control; therefore, women's sexuality is also controlled.

Accessing contraceptive methods is considered to be easy for most women who are married, have a free union relationship, or are single. However, married women represent most of the sample of the respondents (22). Notwithstanding, in this group, women from the parishes of Gasa, Quilloac and Sisid consider that accessing contraceptive methods is difficult or very difficult (see **Figure 4**).

Married women (with elementary school and higher education level) think that the community has to condemn the behavior of single women who use contraceptive methods, as well as they have the perception that this will turn out to be a shame for families. Finally, they consider that the partners of single women who start contraception criticize them. This perception phenomenon is reproduced by women who have a free union relationship. Single women preferred not to answer, which may be associated to the stigma we talked about in the introductory theoretical part of this discussion (see **Figure 5**).

The family planning methods that Cañari indigenous women prefers are: 17 tubal ligation (50%), followed by hormonal injection (16.6%), implant (16.6%), 18 and pill (16.6%), pill (11.1%), and rhythm method (5.55%).

Women between the ages of 39 and 48 have more frequently had tubal ligation (24%), but women between the ages of 29 and 38 (16%) show also this phenomena, while women between the ages of 49 and 59 represent 4%. Young adult women

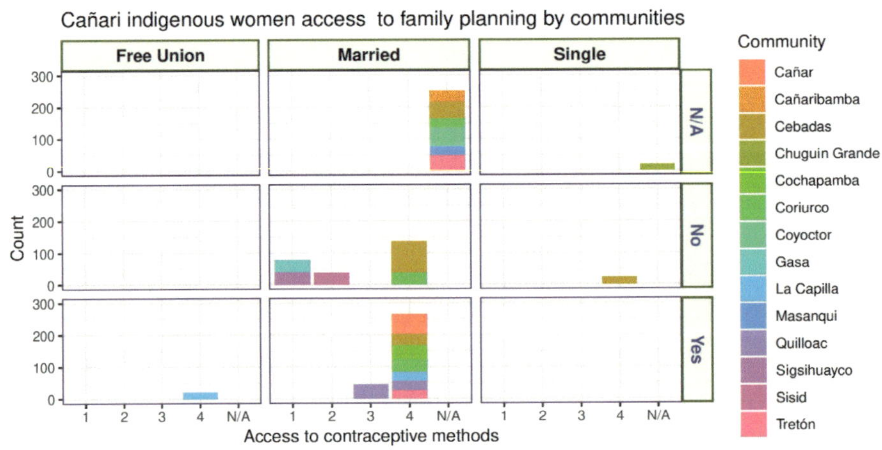

Figure 4.
This figure shows Cañari indigenous women's access to contraceptive methods.

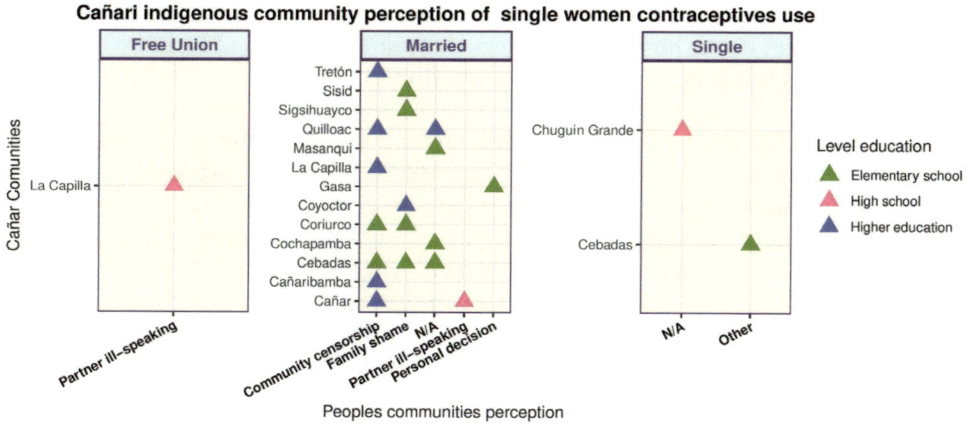

Figure 5.
This figure shows Cañari indigenous communities' perception about single women's use of contraceptives.

Contraceptive methods	Age	Elementary	High school	Higher education	Total
Hormonal injection	19–28	2	1		3
Implant	19–28	1	1	1	3
Pill	19–28			1	1
	39–48			1	1
Rhythm method	29–38	1			1
Tubal ligation	29–38	1		2	3
	39–48		4	1	5
	49–59	1			1
None	19–28	1	1		2
	29–38	1		1	2
	49–59	2		1	3

Table 5.
Prevalent use of contraceptive methods by Cañari indigenous women according to their level of education and age.

(19–28 years old) usually choose methods like hormonal injection, implant and contraceptive pill (28%), probably because they are temporal long-term methods and they still want to have children.

About 28% of Cañari indigenous women do not use any contraceptive method, and this is probably caused by their low level of education, since women in all the age groups (19–28, 29–38, 39–48 and 49–59) that do not use any kind of contraceptive method have elementary or high school education. On the contrary, women who more widely use contraceptives, besides being young (19–28 years old), are those who have elementary school education (see **Table 5**).

The social phenomenon of prevalence of use of contraceptive methods similarly corresponds to women who have elementary school education. On the other hand, in the case of young women who do not use any contraceptive method and have elementary and high school education, the phenomenon is also related to the number of children they have: the higher the level of education they have, the fewer the number of children they have.

3.4 How many children do Cañari indigenous women who have generally had tubal ligation have, how old were they when they decided to have tubal ligation and what is their level of education?

We can see that Cañari indigenous women who have a higher level of education have fewer number of children. Ligation as a method of family planning prevails in the indigenous women of Cañar who have between 5 and 6 children. However, having 8 children in the current era is not prevalent. That is why, only 1 woman had a ligation when having this number of children (see **Figure 6**).

Respondents perceive that both the women they interact with and other women of the community who have undergone tubal ligation consider it to be "very dangerous" (20% and 44.4%). However, other women in these two groups consider tubal ligation to be "very safe" when their close acquaintances have undergone tubal ligation (40%) and also when their close acquaintances have not undergone tubal ligation (33.3%). Similarly, some women consider tubal ligation to be dangerous for their health, harmful for their bodies and the cause of abdominal pain. Finally, they say it weakens their bodies (6.7%), and surveyed women believe that tubal ligation is a sin (6.7%) (see **Figure 7**).

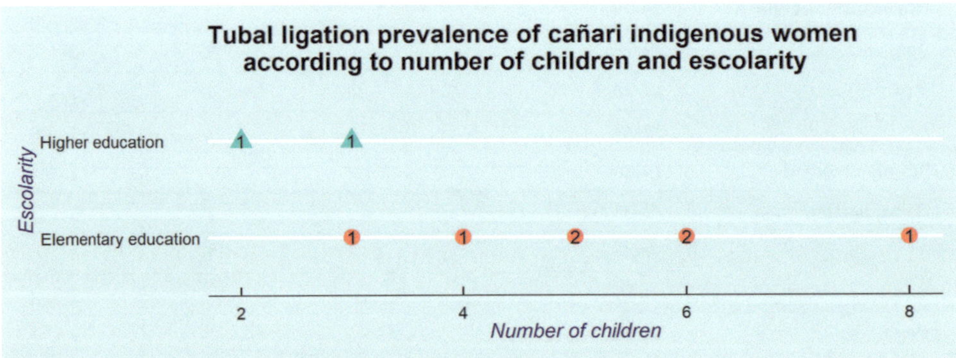

Figure 6.
Prevalent use of tubal ligation by Cañari indigenous women.

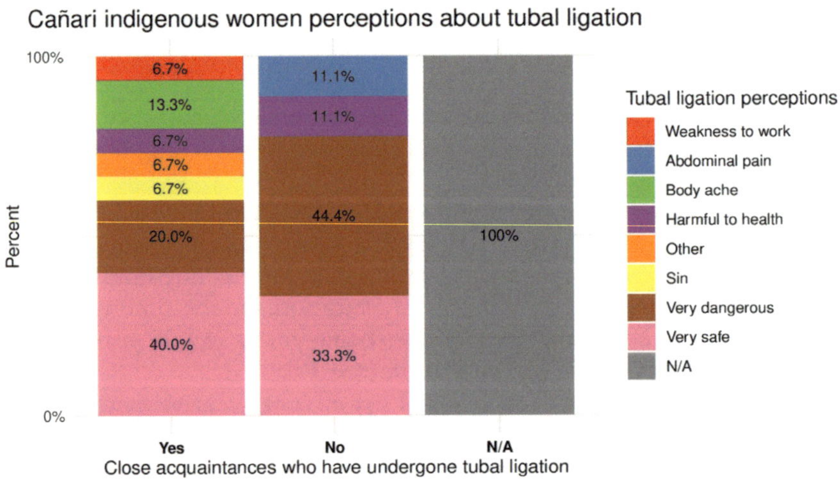

Figure 7.
The figure shows Cañari indigenous women's perception about tubal ligation when their close acquaintances have undergone tubal ligation.

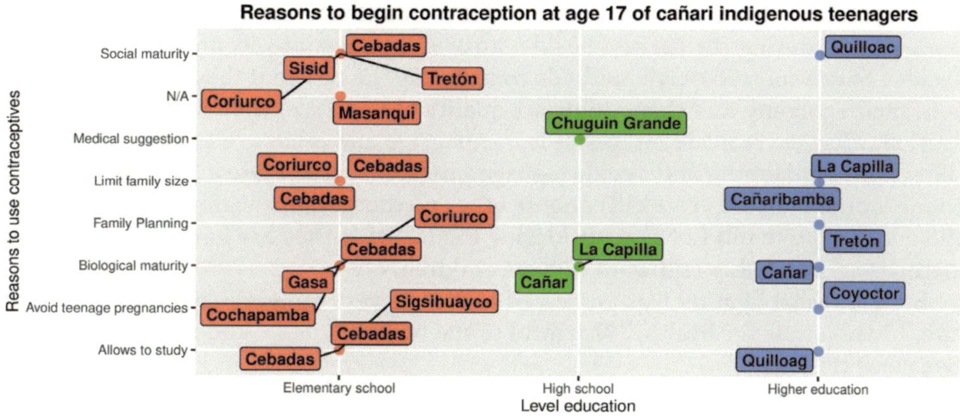

Figure 8.
Respondents with elementary school level education perceive that adolescents at age 17 can, and also should, begin the use of contraceptives because adolescents have biological maturity, adolescents show social maturity, the contraceptives avoid teenage pregnancies and they also allow to study. But respondents with higher education level mostly perceive that adolescents should begin the use of contraceptives at age 17 because of their biological maturity and because the contraceptives limit family size, let family planning, avoid teenage pregnancies and allow to study.

3.5 What is the age to begin the use of contraceptives in Cañari indigenous women, and why?

Cañari indigenous women's perceptions about reasons to begin the use of contraceptives at age 17 in adolescents (see **Figure 8**) is very concerning, because they are too young, and it shows that in this community sexual activity starts very early. This is very dangerous not only because it predisposes them to sexually transmitted infections (STIs), unwanted pregnancy and abortion, but also because their adolescence is reduced, and their adulthood starts early.

4. Conclusions

Based on the results obtained, we can state that the number of children the indigenous women of Cañar have, as it is already known, is connected to their level of education. This research has proven that the higher the number of children these indigenous women have, the fewer the years of education they have (inversely proportional) (see **Table 5**).

The two contraceptive methods that are most widely identified by the indigenous Cañari people between the ages of 19 and 59 are tubal ligation (24%) and hormonal injection (24%), followed by the contraceptive pill (16%), no known method (8%), and, finally, hormonal injection/implant (4%), hormonal injection/tubal ligation (4%), implant (4%), IUD/IUS (4%) and all the rest (4%) (see **Table 3**).

Women having a higher number of children (5–8) are from the rural parishes of Cebadas, Cochapamba, Coriurco and Gasa and have 5 or 6 years of education (elementary school), while single women or women who have a free union relationship have 1 child and come from Chuguin Grande, Cebadas and La Capilla (see **Figure 2**).

Tubal ligation is definitely the preferred contraceptive method (see **Table 4**) by women aged 29–59 (50% of all the family planning methods), including both women having elementary school education (higher number of children) and high school education (fewer number of children). This is defined by the social phenomenon of change of values within this population's cultural system, just as the respondents, during the survey, besides answering questions, confessed that they decided to use contraceptive methods considering the fact that they help to improve both their economy and their children's quality of life. Also, they think that tubal ligation offers several advantages: it is inexpensive and is easy to access, and it allows family planning and avoids teenage pregnancy (see **Figure 3**). However, young women (19–28 years old) choose other methods: hormonal injection, implant and contraceptive pill (28%), considering the fact that they are long-term temporal methods and probably still want to have children.

Besides, tubal ligation was perceived by the surveys as "very dangerous," "very safe," "dangerous for health," "harmful to the body," "causes abdominal pain" and "weakens the body."

It is important to highlight that 28% of Cañari indigenous women do not use any contraceptive method. They are the women who have elementary or high school education. Again, it corresponds to the inversely proportional relationship: the higher the level of education, the fewer the number of children. Choosing natural or traditional contraceptive methods is also connected to "sin," this being the reason that some women value this behavior so as not to break this cultural and religious standard.

In general, accessing contraceptive methods, according to the survey results, is very easy, considering the fact that the Cañari indigenous women who participated in the survey were married (22) (see **Figure 4**). Single women did not want to participate in the survey due to the fact that their marital status limits their answers because they are the target of criticism, as it was indicated in the introductory part of this discussion. For this reason, married women know that their communities condemn the behavior of single women who use contraceptive methods. They also believe that it is a shame for the families of those women, and they think the partners of single women who start using contraceptive methods speak ill of them (see **Figure 5**). The target of criticism that is embodied in single women who use contraceptive methods or participated in the survey is related to shyness or the female stereotype. That is, through the indigenous women's bodies, social control of shyness is manifested in such a way that it becomes the existential basis of shyness. The strong influence of the social control exercised by religion is another important factor. In this study, all the surveys show that these women are Catholic and, as it was stated in the introductory theoretical part of this discussion, the religious component is a system of social control and, consequently, also controls women's sexuality, which is expressed through their bodies.

We need to state that the Cañari culture is marked by a system of values where religion plays the role of socially controlling women's sexual behavior and embodies the stigma of accessing contraceptive methods through a woman's body. This is lived as a set of experiences that modifies these women's access to contraceptive methods and, consequently, to family planning. We can also say that the number of children women having a low level of education have is a factor that determines the occurrence of the previous phenomenon. The fact that some mature adult women undergo tubal ligation is another important factor that needs to be paid attention to. Before 1990 (1987), a record of tubal ligations of women between the ages of 15 and 49 in Ecuador shows the lack of knowledge of this contraceptive method in rural communities; consequently, it was not considered to be a birth control and/or family planning option.

Finally, we also state that there is very concerning the beginning of the contraceptives use in cañari indigenous adolescents (see **Figure 8**) because they start sexual activity very early, and predisposes them to sexually transmitted infections (STIs), unwanted pregnancy and abortion; but, also because their adolescence is reduced, and their adulthood starts before.

Acknowledgements

This project was partially funded by the "Catedra UNESCO UPS Cuenca-Ecuador, Grupo de Investigación en Inteligencia Artificial y Tecnologías de Asistencia (GIATA) CuencaEcuador" and also by "Universidad Politécnica Salesiana."

Conflict of interest

The authors declare no conflict of interest.

Author details

Yaroslava Robles-Bykbaev[1,2]*, Nina Naula[2], Javier Cornejo-Reyes[2,3], Ana Parra[2], Vladimir Robles-Bykbaev[2], Blas Garzón[2] and Jorge Galán[2]

1 Grupo de Investigación en Terapia Celular y Medicina Regenerativa (TCMR), Departamento de Medicina, Universidade da Coruña, Spain

2 GI-IATa, Cátedra UNESCO Tecnologías de apoyo para la Inclusión Educativa, Universidad Politécnica Salesiana, Cuenca, Ecuador

3 Instituto Superior Tecnológico del Azuay (ISTA), Cuenca, Ecuador

*Address all correspondence to: zrobles@ups.edu.ec

References

[1] Özcan M, Beritken Ergin A, Acar Z. Sexual and Reproductive Rights in Turkey: An Owerview. Cokaely, Turkey: Kocaeli Üniversitsi Sosyal Bilimler Dergisi. pp. 122-136

[2] Davis L. Reconocimiento jurídico de los derechos sexuales: Un análisis comparativo con los derechos reproductivos. Sur, Revista Internacional de Direitos Humanos. [online]. 2008;5(8):60-83. DOI: 10.1590/S1806-6445200800 0100004

[3] Organización Mundial de la Salud (OMS). Planificación familiar. [Internet]. 2019. Available from: https://www.who.int/es

[4] Milagros A, Cordero L, Vuttone M. Salud de la mujer indígena: Intervenciones para reducir la muerte materna. Vol. 23. BID, Almería: Editorial Universidad de Almería; 2010

[5] Espinosa, S. Maternidad Indígena: Los derechos, los deseos, las costumbres, en S. Lerner, I. Szasz, Salud Reproductiva y Condiciones de Vida en México, México, D.F.: El Colegio de México. 2008. p. 169

[6] Internacional A. Políticas del cuerpo: manual general sobre la criminalización de la sexualidad y la reproducción. London: Amnesty International Ltd; 2018. p. 52

[7] Pedone C. Madres e Hijas, Rupturas y Continuidades en los Roles de Género en la Migración Ecuatoriana a España. In: Magliano M, Mallimaci A, editors. Las mujeres latinoamericanas y sus migraciones. Córdoba, Argentina: Eduvim; 2016

[8] Baeza P. Maternidad indígena en Colta: un espacio de encuentros y tensiones. Quito: Abya Yala; 2011. p. 17

[9] Weismantel M. Cholas y Pishtacos: Stories of Race and Sex in the Andes. Chicago, USA; University of Chicago Press; 2001. p. 76

[10] Da S, Women K. Gender and Power among Indigenous Peoples of Portuguese Timor. Anuário Antropológico. Brasília: UnB; 2017. pp. 183-205

[11] Cabezas P. Maternidad indígena en Colta: un espacio de encuentros y tensiones. Quito: Abya Yala; 2011. p. 23

[12] Arias M. Determinantes próximos de la fecundidad: Comportamiento reproductivo de las indígenas Chamibida de Antioquia, Colombia. Rio de Janeiro: Cad. Saúde Pública; 2005. pp. 1087-1109. DOI: 10.1590/S0102-311X2005000400011

[13] Urrea F, Posso J. Feminidades, sexualidades y colores de piel: Mujeres negras, indígenas, blancas-mestizas y transgeneristas negras en el suroccidente colombiano. Cali: Programa Editorial Universidad del Valle; 2015

[14] Vázquez V, Flores A. ¿Quién cosecha lo sembrado?: Relaciones de género en un área natural protegida mexicana. México, D.F.: Plaza y Valdes; 2002

[15] Müllauer-Seichter W, Fernández M, Herrera S, Maynar A, Merino M, Vega-Centeno I, et al. Maneras de narrar espacios y tiempos: Ad fontes: Corrientes en Etnohistoria. Vol. 402. Madrid: Editorial Universitaria Ramón Areces; 2012. p. 131

[16] Lirola, M, Carrasco, M, Espinosa, J, Paterna, J. Investigaciones sobre el impacto de la imagen corporal. 2019. ISBN: 978-84-17261-57-3

[17] Csordas T. The Sacred Self: A Cultural Phenomenology of Charismatic

Healing. California: Univesrity of California Press; 1997. pp. 8, 10

[18] Burgos J. La filosofía personalista de Karol Wojtyla. Madrid, Palabra (tesis de maestría). Quito: Universidad Andina Simón Bolívar; 2007. p. 100

[19] Dolezal L. The Body and Shame: Phenomenology, Feminism, and the Socially Shaped Body. London: Lexignton Books; 2015. p. 7

[20] Bouson B. Embodied Shame: Uncovering Female Shame in Contemporary Women's Writings. Vol. 2. New York: Sunny Press; 2010. p. 3

[21] Agudelo J. La planificación familiar Discursos sobre la vida y la sexualidad en Ecuador desde mediados del siglo XX. Quito: Abya Yala; 2017. p. 101

[22] Organización Panamericana de la Salud (OPS) y la Comisión Económica para América Latina y el Caribe (CEPAL). Salud de la población joven indígena en América Latina: un panorama general. Vol. 54. Santiago de Chile: Naciones Unidas; 2011. p. 42

[23] Organización Panamericana de la Salud (OPS). Salud sexual y reproductiva y VIH de los jóvenes y adolescentes indígenas en Bolivia, Ecuador, Guatemala, Nicaragua y Perú. Washington, D.C.: OPS; 2010. p. 61

[24] Ministerio de Salud Pública del Ecuador. Plan Nacional de Salud Sexual y Salud Reproductiva 2017–2021. Quito: MSP; 2017. p. 34

[25] Instituto Nacional de Estadísticas y Censos (INEC). MSP e INEC presentan resultados de Demografía y Salud Sexual y Reproductiva. [Internet]. 2014. Available from: https://www.ecuadorencifras.gob.ec/msp-e-inec-presentan-resultados-de-demografia-y-salud-sexual-y-reproductiva/ [Accessed: 12 December 2019]

[26] Larrea S. Diagnóstico de la situación de la promoción, oferta y demanda de la anticoncepción de emergencia en Loja, Guayas, Pichincha, Esmeraldas y Chimborazo. Quito: Fundación Desafío y Coordinadora Juvenil por la Equidad de Género; 2010. p. 30

[27] Ministerio de Salud Pública del Ecuador (MSP). Situación de Salud de los y las jóvenes indígenas en Ecuador: VIH y Sida y Embarazo en Adolescentes Informe-Ecuador (Español). Quito: MSP; 2010. pp. 40, 51

[28] Instituto Nacional de Estadísticas y Censos (INEC). Comportamiento reproductivo de las mujeres ecuatorianas. Quito: INEC; 2005. p. 30

[29] Instituto Nacional de Estadísticas y Censos (INEC). Las mujeres ecuatorianas que conocen y usan los métodos anticonceptivos. Quito: INEC; 2006. p. 12

[30] Gómez R, Ewerling F, Serruya S, Silveira M, Sanhueza A, Moazzam A, et al. Contraceptive use in Latin America and the Caribbean with a focus on long-acting reversible contraceptives: Prevalence and inequalities in 23 countries. The Lancet. Global Health. 2019. DOI: 10.1016/S2214-109X(18)30481-9

[31] Peláez J. El uso de métodos anticonceptivos en la adolescencia. Rev Cubana Obstet Ginecol. 2016. ISSN: 0138-600X

[32] Rostagnol S. El papel de l@s ginecólog@s en la construcción de los derechos sexuales. In: Uruguay K, Prieto M, editors. Estudios Sobre Sexualidades en América Latina. Quito: FLACSO; 2008. p. 225

[33] Terborgh A, Rosen J, Gálvez R, Terceros W, Bertrand J, Bull S. La planificación familiar entre las poblaciones indígenas de América

Latina. Perspectivas Internacionales en Planificación Familiar. 1996;**4**(11):10

[34] Instituto Nacional de Estadísticas y Censos (INEC). Resultados del Censo 2010 de Población y Vivienda en el Ecuador: fascículo provincial del Cañar [Internet]. 2010. Available from: https://www.ecuadorencifras.gob.ec/wp-content/descargas/Manu-lateral/Resultados-provinciales/canar.pdf

[35] Municipio Intercultural del Cañar. Población [Internet]. 2019. Available from: https://www.canar.gob.ec/gadcanar/index.php/2013-05-20-16-30-14/2013-05-20-16-39-52

[36] Burgos H. La Identidad del Pueblo Cañari: de-construcción de una nación étnica. Quito: Abya Yala; 2003. pp. 33-37

[37] Secretaría Nacional de Planificación y Desarrollo (SENPLADES). Agenda Zonal, ZONA 6-Austro: Provicncias de Azuay, Cañar, y Morona Santiago. 2013–2017. Quito: SENPLADES; 2015. pp. 27, 40, 57

[38] Comisión Económica para América Latina y el Caribe (CEPAL). Población indígena y afroecuatoriana en Ecuador: Diagnóstico sociodemográfico a partir del censo de 2001. Santiago de Chile: Naciones Unidas; 2005. p. 28

[39] Organización Mundial de la Salud Ginebra (OMS). Guía para la Prestación de Servicios. Ginegra: OMS; 1993. p. 6

Section 4

Multiple Gestation

Chapter 5

Multifetal Gestations

Ilkan Kayar

Abstract

In recent years, multiple pregnancy rates have increased significantly. Twin pregnancy rate increased by 76% between 1980 and 2009, from 18.9 to 33.3 in 1000 births. Triplets and high-order multiple pregnancies have increased by 400% in the 1980s and 1990s. Two main reasons of this increase in the incidence of multiple pregnancies are: (1) maternal age at the time of conception, shifting to advanced ages where multiple pregnancies are more common and (2) a more common use of assisted reproductive techniques. The main problem in multiple pregnancies is spontaneous preterm delivery and associated neonatal morbidity and mortality. Although numerous attempts have been made to prolong the gestation period and improve outcomes, none of them have been effective. In this article, the complications encountered in multiple pregnancies will be summarized and evidence-based approaches that can be used in their management will be reported.

Keywords: twins, triplets, monozygotic, dizygotic

1. Introduction

Multiple pregnancy rates have increased significantly in recent years. The twin pregnancy rate increased from 18.9 to 33.3 per 1,000 births between 1980 and 2009, increasing by 76% [1]. Multiple pregnancies with triplets and higher numbers increased by 400% in the 1980s and 1990s [2]. There are two main reasons for this increase in the incidence of multiple pregnancies: (1) Maternal age at the time of conception is shifting to advanced ages with multiple pregnancies and (2) a more common use of assisted reproductive techniques [3].

The main problem encountered in multiple pregnancies is spontaneous preterm labor and associated neonatal morbidity and mortality. Although several attempts have been made to prolong the duration of these pregnancies and improve outcomes, none of them have been effective. In this chapter, the complications encountered in multiple pregnancies will be summarized and evidence-based approaches that can be applied in their management will be reported.

2. Fetal and neonatal morbidity and mortality

Due to complications caused by preterm labor, stillbirth rate in multiple pregnancies is five times higher, and neonatal mortality rate is seven times higher than other pregnancies. A woman with a multiple pregnancy is 6 times more likely to have a preterm delivery and 13 times more likely to give birth before 32 weeks of gestation [4].

In multiple pregnancies, short- and long-term morbidity has also increased. Severe intraventricular hemorrhage and periventricular leukomalacia are two times more common in twins born before 32 weeks of gestation than in single babies born in the same week [5], and this explains the increased rate of cerebral palsy in multiple pregnancies [6].

In multiple pregnancies, still due to the prematurity, health expenses in both antenatal and neonatal periods are higher [7]. The spending made for preterm babies in the year after birth reaches 10 times the spending for full-term babies [8].

3. Chorionicity

Ultrasound is the reliable method to detect multiple pregnancies [9]. Ultrasound shows the number of fetuses, gestational week, chorionicity, and amnionicity. It is very important to detect chorionicity which is best assessed by ultrasound in the first or early second trimester.

Fetal and neonatal mortality and morbidities such as congenital anomaly, prematurity, and intrauterine growth restriction are much more common in monochorionic twins than in dichorionic twins [10, 11]. This also applies to high number of multiple pregnancies; completely monochorionic or monochorionic twin pairs have a higher risk of developing complications compared to trichoricionic triplet pregnancy [12, 13]. Thus, chorionicity should be determined in the late stages of the first trimester or early second trimester for the management of multiple pregnancies and consultancy.

4. Maternal morbidity and mortality

Medical complications such as hyperemesis, gestational diabetes, hypertension, anemia, bleeding, cesarean section, and postpartum depression are more common in women with multiple pregnancies [14–20]. These complications are managed as in singleton pregnancies.

The incidence of hypertensive complications is proportional to the number of fetuses, with 6.5% in singleton pregnancies, 12.7% in twins, and 20% in triplets [21].

In one study, it was found that the risk of developing mild or severe preeclampsia in pregnancies achieved by assisted reproductive techniques was 2.1 times higher than other pregnancies with the same maternal age and parity [22].

Preeclampsia occurs both more frequently (relative risk 2.6) and earlier in twin pregnancies. This results in a higher probability of developing complications such as birth before 35 weeks of gestation (34.5% in twins vs. 6.3% in singles) and ablation of the placenta (4.7% in twins vs. 0.7% in singles) [16]. While preeclampsia is more common in patients with higher-order gestations, it is atypical [23]. If hemolysis, elevated liver enzymes, and low platelet count (HELLP syndrome) occur before term, the patient's referral to the third line will be better for both the mother and the fetus [24].

The incidence of multiple pregnancy increases with age, regardless of assisted reproductive techniques. While the multiple pregnancy rate in women aged under 20 is 16.3 per 1000 live births, this rate is 71.1 per 1000 live births in women over 40 [2]. Regardless of the number of fetuses, obstetric complications such as gestational hypertension, gestational diabetes, and ablation placenta are more common in older women.

5. Effect of assisted reproductive techniques

In the past years, the proliferation of assisted reproductive techniques has led to a serious increase in multiple pregnancy rates [1]. In recent years, there was a decrease in higher-order gestation rates with the limitation of the number of embryos transferred in vitro fertilization (IVF) and the proliferation of embryo reduction. The techniques that cause the most increase in the number of multiple pregnancies are IVF and controlled ovarian hyperstimulation with gonadotropins. According to the most recent data obtained in 2010, 26% of IVF pregnancies result in twins, and 1.3% in higher-order gestations [25].

6. Embryo reduction and selective feticide

Embryo reduction causes a decrease in the risk of spontaneous preterm labor and other obstetric complications with decreased fetal number. In a Cochrane review, it was reported that the pregnancy loss, antenatal complication, preterm birth, low birth weight, and cesarean and neonatal death rates in pregnant women undergoing triplet-to-twin reduction were much lower than in those continuing as triplets and were close to the rates seen in spontaneous twins [26]. Embryo reduction in higher-order gestations also reduces the risk of preeclampsia. In one study, the preeclampsia incidence was 17% in pregnancies with reduction to twins and 30% in pregnancies continuing as triplets [27].

In embryo reduction, the decision of which fetus or fetuses will be treated is determined according to chorionicity and easy accessibility. When one of the monochorionic twin pair is reduced, it is recommended that both monochorionic pair be reduced, since the harmful effects on the other twin are not fully known.

Selective feticide is the reduction of abnormal fetus in a multiple pregnancy. The risk of this procedure is higher compared to embryo reduction, since it is performed at a later gestational week (18th–22nd week instead of 10–12th week) [28]. In higher-order gestations, unwanted loss of healthy fetuses is higher than twins (11.2% vs. 2.4%) [29]. It was observed that gestation period was longer in pregnancies without pregnancy loss [30, 31].

7. Questions and suggestions about clinic

7.1 How to determine chorionicity?

Since fetal risks depend on chorionicity, chorionicity should be determined as early as possible. The ideal period for the determination of chorionicity is late first or early second trimester. In a series, the sensitivity, specificity, and positive and negative predictive values of ultrasound in determining chorionicity before 14 weeks of gestation were 89.8%, 99.5%, 97.8%, and 97.5%, respectively [32], and chorionicity was correctly determined in 95% of cases.

The pregnancy is dichorionic if the ultrasound shows two separate placentas or the gender of fetuses are different. In the case of a single placenta, the most important ultrasound finding used to determine chorionicity is the "twin peak" finding, also known as "lambda" or "delta" sign. This finding shows that there is a triangular shaped protrusion on the chorionic surface of the placenta having the same echogenicity as the placenta and pregnancy is dichorionic [33].

7.2 Is there a test to predict spontaneous preterm labor in multiple pregnancies?

In order to determine the risk of spontaneous preterm labor in asymptomatic pregnant women, many screening methods such as measuring cervical canal length with transvaginal ultrasound, examination of the cervix, fetal fibronectin screening, and home uterus monitoring have been tried. These screening methods are not recommended in asymptomatic women because there is no intervention that can prevent preterm labor in multiple pregnancies that are found to be at high risk for preterm labor [34].

In symptomatic pregnant women, the positive predictive value of fetal fibronectin test alone or short cervical length is low and should not be used for the management of acute symptoms [35]. Although observational studies have shown that fetal fibronectin or cervical canal length precludes the use of unnecessary treatment in singleton pregnancies with preterm labor symptoms, these data have not been proven by randomized controlled trials for either singleton or multiple pregnancies [36–40].

7.3 Are there any interventions to extend the duration of multiple pregnancy?

There is no evidence that interventions such as prophylactic cerclage, routine hospitalization and bed rest, prophylactic tocolysis, and prophylactic pessary reduce neonatal morbidity and mortality. Hence, their use is not recommended in multiple pregnancy.

7.3.1 Prophylactic cerclage

The benefit of prophylactic cerclage in a twin or triplet pregnancy without a history of cervical insufficiency has not been shown [41–43]. In addition, prophylactic cerclage has been reported to increase spontaneous preterm labor by twofold in pregnant women with a short cervical canal on ultrasound (RR, 2.2; 95% [CI], 1.2–4.0) [44, 45]. Therefore, cerclage should be avoided in multiple pregnancies.

7.3.2 Routine hospitalization and bed rest

In a Cochrane review, hospitalization or bed rest has been shown to have no benefit in uncomplicated twin pregnancies [46]. For this reason, routine bed rest should not be recommended to women pregnant with multiples due to the lack of benefit and the risk of thrombosis.

7.3.3 Prophylactic tocolysis

No tocolytic agent should be used for prophylaxis in multiple pregnancies. Maternal complications from tocolysis, such as pulmonary edema, are more common in multiple pregnancies [47, 48]. There are also no data that these drugs reduce the risk of preterm labor or improve neonatal outcomes [49–51]. Oral betamimetics did not reduce preterm delivery, low birth weight, or neonatal mortality in multiple pregnancies compared to placebo [52]. Oral betamimetics are also associated with maternal and fetal cardiac stress and gestational diabetes [53, 54]. It has recently been demonstrated to be associated with adverse maternal cardiovascular events, including death [55].

7.3.4 Prophylactic pessary

There is no scientific evidence that prophylactic cervical pessary reduces the frequency of spontaneous preterm labor or perinatal morbidity in multiple pregnancies. In a recent multicenter randomized controlled study, 813 twin pregnancies from 16 to 20 weeks were randomized [56], and poor perinatal outcome was observed in at least 1 baby of 13% of women treated by Arabin pessary and 14% of other women (RR, 0.98 CI 0.69–1.39). Therefore, the use of prophylactic cervical pessary is not recommended in multiple pregnancies [56].

7.4 Does progesterone treatment reduce the risk of preterm labor in multiple pregnancies?

Progesterone treatment is not recommended in multiple pregnancies since it does not decrease the incidence of preterm labor [57–63]. In one study, it was shown that the use of 17α-hydroxyprogesterone caproate did not reduce neonatal morbidity and prolong pregnancy in triplet pregnancies [61]. In another randomized study, it was shown to significantly increase the rates of fetal loss in the second trimester in triplets [60]. In multiple pregnancies that the cervix was found to be short on transvaginal ultrasound, neither 17α-hydroxyprogesterone caproate nor vaginal progesterone has been demonstrated to be beneficial [64–67].

7.5 How to manage preterm labor in multiple pregnancies?

7.5.1 Tocolytics

Calcium channel blockers or nonsteroidal anti-inflammatory drugs are first-line tocolytic agents. Although there are no large-scale randomized studies conducted only with multiple pregnancies, the current scientific data were obtained from studies involving multiple pregnancies as well as singleton pregnancies [68]. Therefore, in case of an acute preterm labor in multiple pregnancies, short-term tocolysis can be administered up to 48 hours to allow for the administration of corticosteroids.

7.5.2 Corticosteroids

In a Cochrane review, it was concluded that antenatal corticosteroid is beneficial in singleton pregnancies and further studies are required for the outcomes in multiple pregnancies [69]. However, based on its proven benefits in singleton pregnancies, the National Institute of Health recommends the administration of antenatal corticosteroids to pregnant women from 24 to 34 weeks of gestation and who are at risk of giving birth within 7 days, unless there is a contraindication, regardless of the number of fetuses [70, 71].

7.5.3 Magnesium sulfate for fetal neuroprotection

Magnesium sulfate has been shown to reduce the risk and severity of cerebral palsy, regardless of the number of fetuses, at birth before 32 weeks [72–78].

7.6 Prenatal screening in multiple pregnancies

In multiple pregnancies, the probability of one or more fetuses being affected by trisomy is mathematically higher than in singleton pregnancies. For example, maternal age-dependent risk of trisomy in dizygotic twins is twice as much as a singleton pregnancy at the same age [79]. Therefore, the risk of a 33-year-old woman expecting twins is equal to that of a 35-year-old singleton pregnant woman [80].

Aneuploidy screening has many limitations in multiple pregnancies. Serum screening tests in twin or triplet pregnancies are not as sensitive as in singleton pregnancies. The detection rate of trisomy 21 by the second trimester maternal serum screening test in twin pregnancies has been reported to be 63% (71% when both fetuses are affected and 60% when only one is affected) with a false-positive rate of 10.8% [81]. In the first trimester screening test, where maternal age, nuchal transparency, and biochemical markers are evaluated together in twin pregnancies, the detection rate is 75–85% for Down syndrome and 66.7% for trisomy 18, with a false-positive rate of 5% [82–85]. Experience with triplet pregnancies is scarce, but studies show that screening for only nuchal transparency and maternal age is reliable. However, one study has shown that the nuchal transparency above the 95th percentile in monochorionic twin pregnancies predicts 38% of twin-to-twin transfusion syndrome that will develop later, making the interpretation of the first trimester screening results even more complicated in monochorionic pregnancies [86].

Noninvasive prenatal testing can be used for fetal aneuploidy screening, but further data is required to recommend its use in multiple pregnancies [87].

7.7 What are the problems encountered in the prenatal diagnosis of aneuploidy in multiple pregnancies?

Women who wish to have a definitive diagnosis of genetic abnormalities may have an amniocentesis and chorionic villus sampling (CVS). The procedure-related risk of miscarriage for both tests is similar (1–1.8%) and slightly higher compared to singleton pregnancies [88–90]. The main advantage of having CVS is that CVS is performed earlier in pregnancy. However, in multiple pregnancies, some technical difficulties are encountered during these procedures. In approximately 1% of multiple pregnancies, sample for CVS was collected from the wrong fetus [91]. This risk is lower in amniocentesis. To avoid the risk of sampling error, indigo carmine is injected into the first sampled sac after amniocentesis. The absence of dye in the fluid from the second sac proves that sampling was done from two different sacs. Due to the low probability of karyotype being discordant in monochorionic twins, pregnant women may prefer karyotype analysis of a single fetus. Thus, the success of ultrasound in determining chorionicity should be explained to pregnant women.

When aneuploidy is diagnosed, if a fetus is affected, the parents are offered several options, such as termination of the entire pregnancy, selective reduction of the affected fetus, or continuation of pregnancy without any intervention.

7.8 What is the prognosis of multiple pregnancies that are discordant in terms of the size of the fetuses?

Discordant growth in multiple pregnancies is generally defined as a difference of at least 20% between the estimated fetal weights of two fetuses [92, 93]. This rate is calculated by dividing the difference between the weights of the two fetuses by the weight of the larger fetus. It is controversial whether growth discordance leads to negative outcomes in the absence of structural anomaly, aneuploidy, discordant infection, oligohydramnios, or fetal growth restriction. There are studies showing that fetal or neonatal morbidity and mortality do not increase in cases where weight discordance is present but the weight of both fetuses complies with that gestational week [94–97]. However, in multiple pregnancies where the growth of at least one fetus is limited, major neonatal morbidity increases by 7.7 times [98]. In addition, perinatal mortality and morbidity rates were higher in twins with growth restriction than in singleton pregnancies in the same gestational week [99]. In summary, although there is no evidence that neonatal morbidity and mortality increase in twins with discordance only, the risk of adverse perinatal outcomes increases in the presence of an abnormal finding such as fetal growth restriction accompanied by discordance.

7.9 How to manage the death of a fetus?

In the first trimester, spontaneous reduction occurs in one or more fetuses in many of the multiple pregnancies [100]. This likelihood of reduction is proportional to the number of gestational sacs (36% in twins, 53% in triplets, 65% in quadruplets [101]). In the second or third trimester, the death of one or more fetuses is seen in 5% of twins and 17% of triplets [102]. Chorionicity affects the loss rate and helps determine the prognosis and manage the living fetus. In monochorionic-diamniotic twins, the rate of fetal death is higher than in dichorionic-diamniotic twins [103–105]. In fetal deaths after the 14th week of pregnancy, the probability of death of the other twin is 15% in monochorionic twins and 3% in dichorionic twins [105]. The probability of developing neurological abnormalities in the living fetus is 18% in monochorionic twins and 1% in dichorionic twins [106, 107]. Despite these risks, the immediate delivery of the other twin has no benefit [108]. Therefore, in monochorionic twin pregnancies, if one of the fetuses dies before the 34th gestational week, the pregnancy should be managed according to the mother and the living fetus. Unless there is another indication, delivery should not be done before 34th week [109]. The timing of birth should be determined according to the patient and in consultation with those trained in maternal-fetal medicine.

7.10 How to perform antepartum fetal follow-up in dichorionic pregnancies?

After determining chorionicity in the first or early second trimester, the anatomy, size, amount of amniotic fluid, and placenta should be evaluated with ultrasound at 18–22 weeks of gestation. The growth rate of fetuses in uncomplicated twin pregnancies is approximately the same as single pregnancies up to 28–32 weeks [110]. Although there is no scientific evidence suggesting that ultrasound should be performed to evaluate fetal growth after the 20th week, it seems reasonable to monitor dichorionic twin pregnancies without fetal growth restriction or other pregnancy complications every 4–6 weeks with serial ultrasound.

It has not been shown that antepartum tests or umbilical artery Doppler ultrasound improves perinatal outcomes in uncomplicated twin pregnancies [111]. Tests evaluating fetal well-being in dichorionic twins should only be used when there are fetal or maternal complications such as fetal growth restriction.

7.11 How to manage complications caused by monochorionic placentation?

Monochorionic pregnancies should be monitored more closely than dichorionic twins because of the higher risk of complications [112]. Monitoring of pregnancy with serial ultrasound every 2 weeks from the 16th week should be considered [113–115].

7.11.1 Twin-to-twin transfusion syndrome

Twin-to-twin transfusion syndrome develops in approximately 10–15% of monochorionic-diamniotic pregnancies and is due to arteriovenous anastomoses in the monochorionic placenta. It usually occurs in the second trimester and is diagnosed by the presence of oligohydramnios (the largest vertical pocket is smaller than 2 cm) in one sac and polyhydramnios (the largest vertical pocket is larger than 8 cm) in the other sac. A fetal discordance and selective fetal growth restriction due to structural and genetic anomalies or infectious diseases should be ruled out. The benefits of umbilical artery Doppler have not been demonstrated in cases where there is no growth and fluid discordance. The prognosis of twin-to-twin transfusion syndrome varies by the week of gestation and the severity of the syndrome. Staging is based on the Quintero classification system shown in **Table 1**, and treatment with laser coagulation or amnioreduction therapy is frequently used [112, 116].

7.11.2 Monoamniotic twins

The natural incidence of monoamniotic twin pregnancy is one in 10,000, but the incidence may be higher in zona-manipulated IVF pregnancies [117]. Perinatal mortality rates associated with cord complications have been reported as high as 80% [118]. Although the ideal management of these pregnancies is not clearly known, daily fetal heart monitoring in hospital conditions from 24 to 28 weeks of gestation and delivery at 32–34 weeks of gestation are the common practice [118–120].

7.11.3 Rare complications

Acardiac twin pregnancy occurs in 1% of monochorionic pregnancies and is characterized with a fetus that does not have a normally developed heart and brain [121]. This fetus continues to live by the anastomoses in the placenta and the blood supplied by the other fetus (pumping twin). Therefore, the pumping fetus is at risk of cardiac insufficiency, and intrauterine or neonatal loss occurs in nearly half of the cases [122]. This rare condition should be managed by a maternal-fetal medicine specialist experienced in twin pregnancy management.

Conjoined twin is a rare phenomenon, occurring 1 in 50,000–100,000 [123]. After the diagnosis, it should be determined which organs are shared for the prognosis [124]. The survival rate of a conjoined twin detected in the intrauterine period is only 18% even after successful surgery [125].

7.12 What should be the time and mode of delivery in multiple pregnancies?

The time of spontaneous delivery in twin pregnancies is around 36 weeks, and so the complications of prematurity are an important risk [126]. Perinatal mortality increases again after 38 weeks of gestation [127]. Accordingly the time of delivery for uncomplicated twin pregnancies would be reasonable [108]:

a. At 38 weeks in dichorionic diamniotic twins without complications

b. From 34 to 37 6/7 weeks in monochorionic-diamniotic pregnancies without complications

c. From 32 to 34 weeks in monoamniotic pregnancies without complications

The ideal mode of delivery varies by the type of twin pregnancy, the presentation of the fetuses, the gestational week, and the experience of the delivering physician. Twin pregnancy alone is not an indication of cesarean section [128]. In monoamniotic pregnancies only, cesarean delivery is required to avoid cord complications that may develop in the other fetus during the birth of the first fetus [118].

In a recently published randomized controlled study, no difference was reported between planned cesarean and planned vaginal delivery in terms of fetal and neonatal death or severe neonatal morbidity between 32 and 38 6/7 weeks of gestation in twin pregnancies with cephalic presentation of the first fetus [129]. Therefore, in diamniotic twin pregnancies with cephalic presentation of the first fetus after the 32nd gestational week, vaginal delivery appears to be a logical option, regardless of the presentation of the second fetus, provided that the obstetrician is experienced in internal podalic version and vaginal breech delivery [130].

The ideal delivery method in higher-order multiple pregnancies is not known. In small observational studies, there was no significant difference between planned vaginal delivery and planned cesarean delivery with the cephalic presentation of the first fetus in uncomplicated triplet pregnancies. Therefore, planned vaginal delivery may be considered in these pregnancies if obstetrician is experienced [131–133]. Vaginal delivery can be attempted in twin pregnancies with a previous history of cesarean section with a single lower transverse incision and without any contraindications for vaginal delivery [134–138]. Internal fetal manipulation or emergency cesarean section may be required during delivery. Women with multiple pregnancies are at risk for atony, postpartum bleeding, and emergency hysterectomy [139]. The administration of neuroaxial analgesia facilitates operative vaginal delivery, external or internal cephalic version, and total breech extraction in multiple pregnancies [130].

Stage 1. Monochorionic-diamniotic gestation with oligohydramnios (MVP less than 2 cm) and polyhydramnios (MVP greater than 8 cm)
Stage 2. Absent (empty) bladder in donor
Stage 3. Abnormal Doppler ultrasonography findings*
Stage 4. Hydrops
Stage 5. Death of one or both twins

Abbreviation: MVP, maximum vertical pocket. Data from [140].
**Defined as the presence of one or more of the following: umbilical artery absent or reversed diastolic flow; ductus venosus absent or reversed diastolic flow; or umbilical vein pulsatile flow.*

Table 1.
Staging of twin-to-twin transfusion syndrome.

8. Summary of findings and recommendations

A. Recommendations based on reliable scientific data (with evidence level A)

- No tocolytic agent is recommended for prophylactic use in multiple pregnancies.
- Treatment with progesterone does not reduce the incidence of spontaneous preterm delivery in twin and triplet pregnancies.

B. Recommendations based on limited scientific data (with evidence level B)

- Chorionicity should be determined in the late stages of the first trimester or in the early stages of the second trimester due to complications of monochorionicity.
- Since prophylactic tocolysis, prophylactic cerclage, prophylactic pessary, routine hospitalization, and bed rest have not been shown to reduce neonatal

morbidity and mortality, these practices are not recommended in multiple pregnancies.

- Magnesium sulfate has been shown to reduce the risk and severity of cerebral palsy, regardless of the number of fetuses, at birth before 32 weeks.

- In women with a previous history of cesarean section with a transverse incision to the lower segment, vaginal delivery can be attempted unless there is another contraindication.

- In pregnancies in which the number of fetuses is reduced from three to two with embryo reduction, pregnancy loss, antenatal complications, preterm delivery, low birth weight, and cesarean and neonatal mortality rates are lower than in pregnancies continuing as triplets and are similar to spontaneous twin pregnancies.

- Unless there are contraindications, a cycle of antenatal corticosteroid should be administered to women pregnant with multiples from 24 to 34 weeks of gestation and who are expected to give birth within 7 days regardless of the number of fetuses.

C. Recommendations based on expert opinion (with evidence level C)

- Delivery in uncomplicated monoamniotic twins should be at 32–34 weeks of gestation.

- In diamniotic twin pregnancies over 32 0/7 weeks with cephalic presentation of the first fetus, vaginal delivery appears to be a logical option, regardless of the presentation of the second fetus, provided that the obstetrician is experienced in internal podalic version and vaginal breech delivery.

- Women with multiple pregnancies are candidates for routine aneuploidy screening regardless of age.

- Administration of neuroaxial (epidural) analgesia in multiple pregnancies facilitates operative vaginal delivery, external or internal cephalic version, and total breech extraction.

- Monoamniotic twin pregnancies should be delivered by cesarean.

DOI: http://dx.doi.org/10.5772/intechopen.92050

Author details

Ilkan Kayar
Department of Obstetrics and Gynecology, Osmaniye State Hospital, Osmaniye, Turkey

*Address all correspondence to: ilkankayar@gmail.com

References

[1] Martin JA, Hamilton BE, Osterman MJ. Three decades of twin births in the United States, 1980-2009. NCHS Data Brief. 2012;**80**:1-8

[2] Martin JA, Hamilton BE, Ventura SJ, Osterman MJ, Kirmeyer S, Mathews TJ, et al. Births: Final data for 2009. National Vital Statistics Reports. 2011;**60**:1-70

[3] Blondel B, Kaminski M. Trends in the occurrence, determinants, and consequences of multiple births. Seminars in Perinatology. 2002;**26**:239-249

[4] Scher AI, Petterson B, Blair E, Ellenberg JH, Grether JK, Haan E, et al. The risk of mortality or cerebral palsy in twins: A collaborative population-based study. Pediatric Research. 2002;**52**:671-681

[5] Rettwitz-Volk W, Tran TM, Veldman A. Cerebral morbidity in preterm twins. The Journal of Maternal-Fetal & Neonatal Medicine. 2003;**13**:218-223

[6] Yokoyama Y, Shimizu T, Hayakawa K. Prevalence of cerebral palsy in twins, triplets and quadruplets. International Journal of Epidemiology. 1995;**24**:943-948

[7] Bromer JG, Ata B, Seli M, Lockwood CJ, Seli E. Preterm deliveries that result from multiple pregnancies associated with assisted reproductive technologies in the USA: A cost analysis. Current Opinion in Obstetrics & Gynecology. 2011;**23**:168-173

[8] Institute of Medicine. Preterm Birth: Causes, Consequences, and Prevention. Washington, DC: National Academies Press; 2007

[9] LeFevre ML, Bain RP, Ewigman BG, Frigoletto FD, Crane JP, McNellis D. A randomized trial of prenatal ultrasonographic screening: Impact on maternal management and outcome. RADIUS (Routine Antenatal Diagnostic Imaging with Ultrasound) Study Group. American Journal of Obstetrics and Gynecology. 1993;**169**:483-489

[10] Geipel A, Berg C, Katalinic A, Plath H, Hansmann M, Germer U, et al. Prenatal diagnosis and obstetric outcomes in triplet pregnancies in relation to chorionicity. BJOG. 2005;**112**:554-558

[11] Glinianaia SV, Obeysekera MA, Sturgiss S, Bell R. Stillbirth and neonatal mortality in monochorionic and dichorionic twins: A population-based study. Human Reproduction. 2011;**26**:2549-2557

[12] Bajoria R, Ward SB, Adegbite AL. Comparative study of perinatal outcome of dichorionic and trichorionic iatrogenic triplets. American Journal of Obstetrics and Gynecology. 2006;**194**:415-424

[13] Kawaguchi H, Ishii K, Yamamoto R, Hayashi S, Mitsuda N. Perinatal death of triplet pregnancies by chorionicity. Perinatal Research Network Group in Japan. American Journal of Obstetrics and Gynecology. 2013;**209**:36.e1-36.e7

[14] Sivan E, Maman E, Homko CJ, Lipitz S, Cohen S, Schiff E. Impact of fetal reduction on the incidence of gestational diabetes. Obstetrics and Gynecology. 2002;**99**:91-94

[15] Schwartz DB, Daoud Y, Zazula P, Goyert G, Bronsteen R, Wright D, et al. Gestational diabetes mellitus: Metabolic and blood glucose parameters in singleton versus twin pregnancies. American Journal of Obstetrics and Gynecology. 1999;**181**:912-914

[16] Sibai BM, Hauth J, Caritis S, Lindheimer MD, MacPherson C, Klebanoff M, et al. Hypertensive disorders in twin versus singleton gestations. National Institute of Child Health and Human Development Network of Maternal-Fetal Medicine Units. American Journal of Obstetrics and Gynecology. 2000;**182**:938-942

[17] Luke B, Brown MB. Contemporary risks of maternal morbidity and adverse outcomes with increasing maternal age and plurality. Fertility and Sterility. 2007;**88**:283-293

[18] Conde-Agudelo A, Belizan JM, Lindmark G. Maternal morbidity and mortality associated with multiple gestations. Obstetrics and Gynecology. 2000;**95**:899-904

[19] Sheard C, Cox S, Oates M, Ndukwe G, Glazebrook C. Impact of a multiple, IVF birth on post-partum mental health: A composite analysis. Human Reproduction. 2007;**22**:2058-2065

[20] Bailit JL. Hyperemesis gravidarium: Epidemiologic findings from a large cohort. American Journal of Obstetrics and Gynecology. 2005;**193**:811-814

[21] Day MC, Barton JR, O'Brien JM, Istwan NB, Sibai BM. The effect of fetal number on the development of hypertensive conditions of pregnancy. Obstetrics and Gynecology. 2005;**106**:927-931

[22] Lynch A, McDuffie R Jr, Murphy J, Faber K, Orleans M. Preeclampsia in multiple gestation: The role of assisted reproductive technologies. Obstetrics and Gynecology. 2002;**99**:445-451

[23] Hardardottir H, Kelly K, Bork MD, Cusick W, Campbell WA, Rodis JF. Atypical presentation of preeclampsia in high-order multifetal gestations. Obstetrics and Gynecology. 1996;**87**:370-374

[24] Sibai BM. Diagnosis, controversies, and management of the syndrome of hemolysis, elevated liver enzymes, and low platelet count. Obstetrics and Gynecology. 2004;**103**:981-991

[25] Society for Assisted Reproductive Technology. Clinic Summary Report: All SART Member Clinics. Available from: https://www.sartcorsonline.com/rptCSR_PublicMultYear.aspx?ClinicPKID=0 [Accessed: 05 February 2014]

[26] Dodd JM, Crowther CA. Reduction of the number of fetuses for women with a multiple pregnancy. Cochrane Database of Systematic Reviews. 2012;(10):CD003932. DOI: 10.1002/14651858.CD003932.pub3

[27] Smith-Levitin M, Kowalik A, Birnholz J, Skupski DW, Hutson JM, Chervenak FA, et al. Selective reduction of multifetal pregnancies to twins improves outcome over nonreduced triplet gestations. American Journal of Obstetrics and Gynecology. 1996;**175**:878-882

[28] Berkowitz RL, Stone JL, Eddleman KA. One hundred consecutive cases of selective termination of an abnormal fetus in a multifetal gestation. Obstetrics and Gynecology. 1997;**90**:606-610

[29] Eddleman KA, Stone JL, Lynch L, Berkowitz RL. Selective termination of anomalous fetuses in multifetal pregnancies: Two hundred cases at a single center. American Journal of Obstetrics and Gynecology. 2002;**187**:1168-1172

[30] Lust A, De Catte L, Lewi L, Deprest J, Loquet P, Devlieger R. Monochorionic and dichorionic twin pregnancies discordant for fetal anencephaly: A systematic review of prenatal management options. Prenatal Diagnosis. 2008;**28**:275-279

[31] Lynch L, Berkowitz RL, Stone J, Alvarez M, Lapinski R. Preterm delivery after selective termination in twin pregnancies. Obstetrics and Gynecology. 1996;**87**:366-369

[32] Lee YM, Cleary-Goldman J, Thaker HM, Simpson LL. Antenatal sonographic prediction of twin chorionicity. American Journal of Obstetrics and Gynecology. 2006;**195**:863-867

[33] Finberg HJ. The "twin peak" sign: Reliable evidence of dichorionic twinning. Journal of Ultrasound in Medicine. 1992;**11**:571-577

[34] Reichmann JP. Home uterine activity monitoring: An evidence review of its utility in multiple gestations. The Journal of Reproductive Medicine. 2009;**54**:559-562

[35] Berghella V, Hayes E, Visintine J, Baxter JK. Fetal fibronectin testing for reducing the risk of preterm birth. Cochrane Database of Systematic Reviews. 2008;(4):CD006843. DOI: 10.1002/14651858.CD006843.pub2

[36] Joffe GM, Jacques D, Bemis-Heys R, Burton R, Skram B, Shelburne P. Impact of the fetal fibronectin assay on admissions for preterm labor. American Journal of Obstetrics and Gynecology. 1999;**180**:581-586

[37] Giles W, Bisits A, Knox M, Madsen G, Smith R. The effect of fetal fibronectin testing on admissions to a tertiary maternal-fetal medicine unit and cost savings. American Journal of Obstetrics and Gynecology. 2000;**182**:439-442

[38] Grobman WA, Welshman EE, Calhoun EA. Does fetal fibronectin use in the diagnosis of preterm labor affect physician behavior and health care costs? A randomized trial. American Journal of Obstetrics and Gynecology. 2004;**191**:235-240

[39] Ness A, Visintine J, Ricci E, Berghella V. Does knowledge of cervical length and fetal fibronectin affect management of women with threatened preterm labor? A randomized trial. American Journal of Obstetrics and Gynecology. 2007;**197**:426.e1-426.e7

[40] Plaut MM, Smith W, Kennedy K. Fetal fibronectin: The impact of a rapid test on the treatment of women with preterm labor symptoms. American Journal of Obstetrics and Gynecology. 2003;**188**:1588-1593 discussion 1593-5

[41] Dor J, Shalev J, Mashiach S, Blankstein J, Serr DM. Elective cervical suture of twin pregnancies diagnosed ultrasonically in the first trimester following induced ovulation. Gynecologic and Obstetric Investigation. 1982;**13**:55-60

[42] Rebarber A, Roman AS, Istwan N, Rhea D, Stanziano G. Prophylactic cerclage in the management of triplet pregnancies. American Journal of Obstetrics and Gynecology. 2005;**193**:1193-1196

[43] Moragianni VA, Aronis KN, Craparo FJ. Biweekly ultrasound assessment of cervical shortening in triplet pregnancies and the effect of cerclage placement. Ultrasound in Obstetrics & Gynecology. 2011;**37**:617-618

[44] Berghella V, Odibo AO, To MS, Rust OA, Althuisius SM. Cerclage for short cervix on ultrasonography: Meta-analysis of trials using individual patient-level data. Obstetrics and Gynecology. 2005;**106**:181-189

[45] Roman AS, Saltzman DH, Fox N, Klauser CK, Istwan N, Rhea D, et al. Prophylactic cerclage in the management of twin pregnancies. American Journal of Perinatology. 2013;**30**:751-754

[46] Crowther CA, Han S. Hospitalisation and bed rest for multiple pregnancy. Cochrane Database of Systematic Reviews. 2010;(7):CD000110. DOI: 10.1002/14651858.CD000110.pub2

[47] Wilkins IA, Lynch L, Mehalek KE, Berkowitz GS, Berkowitz RL. Efficacy and side effects of magnesium sulfate and ritodrine as tocolytic agents. American Journal of Obstetrics and Gynecology. 1988;**159**:685-689

[48] Samol JM, Lambers DS. Magnesium sulfate tocolysis and pulmonary edema: The drug or the vehicle? American Journal of Obstetrics and Gynecology. 2005;**192**:1430-1432

[49] Cetrulo CL, Freeman RK. Ritodrine HCL for the prevention of premature labor in twin pregnancies. Acta Geneticae Medicae et Gemellologiae. 1976;**25**:321-324

[50] O'Leary JA. Prophylactic tocolysis of twins. American Journal of Obstetrics and Gynecology. 1986;**154**:904-905

[51] Ashworth MF, Spooner SF, Verkuyl DA, Waterman R, Ashurst HM. Failure to prevent preterm labour and delivery in twin pregnancy using prophylactic oral salbutamol. British Journal of Obstetrics and Gynaecology. 1990;**97**:878-882

[52] Yamasmit W, Chaithongwongwatthana S, Tolosa JE, Limpongsanurak S, Pereira L, Lumbiganon P. Prophylactic oral betamimetics for reducing preterm birth in women with a twin pregnancy. Cochrane Database of Systematic Reviews. 2012;(9):CD004733. DOI: 10.1002/14651858.CD004733.pub3

[53] Fletcher SE, Fyfe DA, Case CL, Wiles HB, Upshur JK, Newman RB. Myocardial necrosis in a newborn after long-term maternal subcutaneous terbutaline infusion for suppression of preterm labor. American Journal of Obstetrics and Gynecology. 1991;**165**:1401-1404

[54] Gabriel R, Harika G, Saniez D, Durot S, Quereux C, Wahl P. Prolonged intravenous ritodrine therapy: A comparison between multiple and singleton pregnancies. European Journal of Obstetrics, Gynecology, and Reproductive Biology. 1994;**57**:65-71

[55] Food and Drug Administration. FDA Drug Safety Communication: New Warnings against Use of Terbutaline to Treat Preterm Labor. Silver Spring (MD): FDA; 2011. Available from: http://www.fda.gov/drugs/drugsafety/ucm243539.htm [Accessed: 31 January 2014]

[56] Liem S, Schuit E, Hegeman M, Bais J, de Boer K, Bloemenkamp K, et al. Cervical pessaries for prevention of preterm birth in women with a multiple pregnancy (ProTWIN): A multicentre, open-label randomised controlled trial. Lancet. 2013;**382**:1341-1349

[57] Rouse DJ, Caritis SN, Peaceman AM, Sciscione A, Thom EA, Spong CY, et al. A trial of 17 alpha-hydroxyprogesterone caproate to prevent prematurity in twins. National Institute of Child Health and Human Development Maternal Fetal Medicine Units Network. The New England Journal of Medicine. 2007;**357**:454-461

[58] Norman JE, Mackenzie F, Owen P, Mactier H, Hanretty K, Cooper S, et al. Progesterone for the prevention of preterm birth in twin pregnancy (STOPPIT): A randomised, double-blind, placebo-controlled study and meta-analysis. Lancet. 2009;**373**:2034-2040

[59] Combs CA, Garite T, Maurel K, Das A, Porto M. 17-hydroxyprogesterone caproate for twin pregnancy: A double-blind, randomized clinical trial. Obstetrix Collaborative

Research Network. American Journal of Obstetrics and Gynecology. 2011;**204**:221.e1-221.e8

[60] Combs CA, Garite T, Maurel K, Das A, Porto M. Failure of 17-hydroxyprogesterone to reduce neonatal morbidity or prolong triplet pregnancy: A double-blind, randomized clinical trial. Obstetrix Collaborative Research Network [published erratum appears in Am J Obstet Gynecol 2011;204:166]. American Journal of Obstetrics and Gynecology. 2010;**203**:248.e1-248.e9

[61] Caritis SN, Rouse DJ, Peaceman AM, Sciscione A, Momirova V, Spong CY, et al. Prevention of preterm birth in triplets using 17 alpha-hydroxyprogesterone caproate: A randomized controlled trial. Eunice Kennedy Shriver National Institute of Child Health and Human Development (NICHD), Maternal-Fetal Medicine Units Network (MFMU). Obstetrics and Gynecology. 2009;**113**:285-292

[62] Durnwald CP, Momirova V, Rouse DJ, Caritis SN, Peaceman AM, Sciscione A, et al. Second trimester cervical length and risk of preterm birth in women with twin gestations treated with 17-alpha hydroxyprogesterone caproate. Eunice Kennedy Shriver National Institute of Child Health and Human Development Maternal-Fetal Medicine Units Network. The Journal of Maternal-Fetal & Neonatal Medicine. 2010;**23**:1360-1364

[63] Wood S, Ross S, Tang S, Miller L, Sauve R, Brant R. Vaginal progesterone to prevent preterm birth in multiple pregnancy: A randomized controlled trial. Journal of Perinatal Medicine. 2012. DOI: 10.1515/jpm-2012-0057 (Level I)

[64] Fonseca EB, Celik E, Parra M, Singh M, Nicolaides KH. Progesterone and the risk of preterm birth among women with a short cervix. Fetal Medicine Foundation Second Trimester Screening Group. The New England Journal of Medicine. 2007;**357**:462-469

[65] Romero J, Rebarber A, Saltzman DH, Schwartz R, Peress D, Fox NS. The prediction of recurrent preterm birth in patients on 17-alpha-hydroxyprogesterone caproate using serial fetal fibronectin and cervical length. American Journal of Obstetrics and Gynecology. 2012;**207**:51.e1-51.e5

[66] Senat MV, Porcher R, Winer N, Vayssiere C, Deruelle P, Capelle M, et al. Prevention of preterm delivery by 17 alpha-hydroxyprogesterone caproate in asymptomatic twin pregnancies with a short cervix: A randomized controlled trial. Groupe de Recherche en Obstetrique et Gynecologie. American Journal of Obstetrics and Gynecology. 2013;**208**:194.e1-194.e8

[67] Serra V, Perales A, Meseguer J, Parrilla JJ, Lara C, Bellver J, et al. Increased doses of vaginal progesterone for the prevention of preterm birth in twin pregnancies: A randomised controlled double-blind multicentre trial. BJOG. 2013;**120**:50-57

[68] Haas DM, Quinney SK, Clay JM, Renbarger JL, Hebert MF, Clark S, et al. Nifedipine pharmacokinetics are influenced by CYP3A5 genotype when used as a preterm labor tocolytic. Obstetric-Fetal Pharmacology Research Units Network. American Journal of Perinatology. 2013;**30**:275-281

[69] Roberts D, Dalziel SR. Antenatal corticosteroids for accelerating fetal lung maturation for women at risk of preterm birth. Cochrane Database of Systematic Reviews. 2006;(3):CD004454. DOI: 10.1002/14651858.CD004454.pub2

[70] Effect of corticosteroids for fetal maturation on perinatal outcomes. NIH Consens Statement. 1994;**12**(2):1-24

[71] Antenatal corticosteroid therapy for fetal maturation. Committee Opinion No. 677. American College of Obstetricians and Gynecologists. Obstetrics and Gynecology. 2016;**128**:e187-e194

[72] Crowther CA, Hiller JE, Doyle LW, Haslam RR. Effect of magnesium sulfate given for neuroprotection before preterm birth: A randomized controlled trial. Australasian Collaborative Trial of Magnesium Sulphate (ACTOMg SO4) Collaborative Group. JAMA. 2003;**290**:2669-2676

[73] Marret S, Marpeau L, Zupan-Simunek V, Eurin D, Leveque C, Hellot MF, et al. Magnesium sulphate given before very-preterm birth to protect infant brain: The randomised controlled PREMAG trial. PREMAG trial group. BJOG. 2007;**114**:310-318

[74] Rouse DJ, Hirtz DG, Thom E, Varner MW, Spong CY, Mercer BM, et al. A randomized, controlled trial of magnesium sulfate for the prevention of cerebral palsy. Eunice Kennedy Shriver NICHD Maternal-Fetal Medicine Units Network. The New England Journal of Medicine. 2008;**359**:895-905

[75] Doyle LW, Crowther CA, Middleton P, Marret S, Rouse D. Magnesium sulphate for women at risk of preterm birth for neuroprotection of the fetus. Cochrane Database of Systematic Reviews. 2009;(1): CD004661. DOI: 10.1002/14651858. CD004661.pub3

[76] Conde-Agudelo A, Romero R. Antenatal magnesium sulfate for the prevention of cerebral palsy in preterm infants less than 34 weeks' gestation: A systematic review and metaanalysis. American Journal of Obstetrics and Gynecology. 2009;**200**:595-609

[77] Costantine MM, Weiner SJ. Effects of antenatal exposure to magnesium sulfate on neuroprotection and mortality in preterm infants: A meta-analysis. Eunice Kennedy Shriver National Institute of Child Health and Human Development Maternal-Fetal Medicine Units Network. Obstetrics and Gynecology. 2009;**114**:354-364

[78] Magnesium sulfate before anticipated preterm birth for neuroprotection. Committee Opinion No. 455. American College of Obstetricians and Gynecologists. Obstetrics and Gynecology. 2010;**115**:669-671

[79] Meyers C, Adam R, Dungan J, Prenger V. Aneuploidy in twin gestations: When is maternal age advanced? Obstetrics and Gynecology. 1997;**89**:248-251

[80] Rodis JF, Egan JF, Craffey A, Ciarleglio L, Greenstein RM, Scorza WE. Calculated risk of chromosomal abnormalities in twin gestations. Obstetrics and Gynecology. 1990;**76**:1037-1041

[81] Garchet-Beaudron A, Dreux S, Leporrier N, Oury JF, Muller F. Second-trimester Down syndrome maternal serum marker screening: A prospective study of 11 040 twin pregnancies. ABA Study Group, Clinical Study Group. Prenatal Diagnosis. 2008;**28**:1105-1109

[82] Bush MC, Malone FD. Down syndrome screening in twins. Clinics in Perinatology. 2005;**32**:373-386 vi

[83] Chasen ST, Perni SC, Kalish RB, Chervenak FA. First trimester risk assessment for trisomies 21 and 18 in twin pregnancy. American Journal of Obstetrics and Gynecology. 2007;**197**:374.e1-374.e3

[84] Sebire NJ, Snijders RJ, Hughes K, Sepulveda W, Nicolaides KH. Screening for trisomy 21 in twin pregnancies by maternal age and fetal nuchal translucency thickness at 10-14 weeks of gestation. British Journal of Obstetrics and Gynaecology. 1996;**103**:999-1003

[85] Sepulveda W, Wong AE, Casasbuenas A. Nuchal translucency and nasal bone in first-trimester ultrasound screening for aneuploidy in multiple pregnancies. Ultrasound in Obstetrics & Gynecology. 2009;**33**:152-156

[86] Sebire NJ, D'Ercole C, Hughes K, Carvalho M, Nicolaides KH. Increased nuchal translucency thickness at 10-14 weeks of gestation as a predictor of severe twin-to-twin transfusion syndrome. Ultrasound in Obstetrics & Gynecology. 1997;**10**:86-89

[87] Noninvasive prenatal testing for fetal aneuploidy. Committee Opinion No. 545. American College of Obstetricians and Gynecologists. Obstetrics and Gynecology. 2012;**120**:1532-1534

[88] Agarwal K, Alfirevic Z. Pregnancy loss after chorionic villus sampling and genetic amniocentesis in twin pregnancies: A systematic review. Ultrasound in Obstetrics & Gynecology. 2012;**40**:128-134

[89] Simonazzi G, Curti A, Farina A, Pilu G, Bovicelli L, Rizzo N. Amniocentesis and chorionic villus sampling in twin gestations: Which is the best sampling technique? American Journal of Obstetrics and Gynecology. 2010;**202**:365.e1-365.e5

[90] Cahill AG, Macones GA, Stamilio DM, Dicke JM, Crane JP, Odibo AO. Pregnancy loss rate after mid-trimester amniocentesis in twin pregnancies. American Journal of Obstetrics and Gynecology. 2009;**200**:257.e1-257.e6

[91] Eddleman KA, Stone JL, Lynch L, Berkowitz RL. Chorionic villus sampling before multifetal pregnancy reduction. American Journal of Obstetrics and Gynecology. 2000;**183**:1078-1081

[92] Talbot GT, Goldstein RF, Nesbitt T, Johnson JL, Kay HH. Is size discordancy an indication for delivery of preterm twins? American Journal of Obstetrics and Gynecology. 1997;**177**:1050-1054

[93] Breathnach FM, McAuliffe FM, Geary M, Daly S, Higgins JR, Dornan J, et al. Definition of intertwin birth weight discordance. Obstetrics & Gynecology. 2011;**118**(1):94-103. DOI: 10.1097/AOG.0b013e31821fd208

[94] Lopriore E, Slaghekke F, Vandenbussche FP, Middeldorp JM, Walther FJ, Oepkes D. Cerebral injury in monochorionic twins with selective intrauterine growth restriction and/or birthweight discordance. American Journal of Obstetrics and Gynecology. 2008;**199**:628.e1-628.e5

[95] Appleton C, Pinto L, Centeno M, Clode N, Cardoso C, Graca LM. Near term twin pregnancy: Clinical relevance of weight discordance at birth. Journal of Perinatal Medicine. 2007;**35**:62-66

[96] Cohen SB, Elizur SE, Goldenberg M, Beiner M, Novikov I, Mashiach S, et al. Outcome of twin pregnancies with extreme weight discordancy. American Journal of Perinatology. 2001;**18**:427-432

[97] Kilic M, Aygun C, Kaynar-Tuncel E, Kucukoduk S. Does birth weight discordance in preterm twins affect neonatal outcome? Journal of Perinatology. 2006;**26**:268-272

[98] Yinon Y, Mazkereth R, Rosentzweig N, Jarus-Hakak A, Schiff E, Simchen MJ. Growth restriction as a determinant of outcome in preterm discordant twins. Obstetrics and Gynecology. 2005;**105**:80-84

[99] Odibo AO, McDonald RE, Stamilio DM, Ural SH, Macones GA. Perinatal outcomes in growth-restricted twins compared with age-matched growth-restricted singletons.

American Journal of Perinatology. 2005;**22**:269-273

[100] Landy HJ, Keith LG. The vanishing twin: A review. Human Reproduction Update. 1998;**4**:177-183

[101] Dickey RP, Taylor SN, Lu PY, Sartor BM, Storment JM, Rye PH, et al. Spontaneous reduction of multiple pregnancy: Incidence and effect on outcome. American Journal of Obstetrics and Gynecology. 2002;**186**:77-83

[102] D'Alton ME, Simpson LL. Syndromes in twins. Seminars in Perinatology. 1995;**19**:375-386

[103] Lee YM, Wylie BJ, Simpson LL, D'Alton ME. Twin chorionicity and the risk of stillbirth [published erratum appears in Obstet Gynecol 2008;111:1217]. Obstetrics and Gynecology. 2008;**111**:301-308

[104] Morikawa M, Yamada T, Yamada T, Sato S, Cho K, Minakami H. Prospective risk of stillbirth: Monochorionic diamniotic twins vs. dichorionic twins. Journal of Perinatal Medicine. 2012;**40**:245-249

[105] Danon D, Sekar R, Hack KE, Fisk NM. Increased stillbirth in uncomplicated monochorionic twin pregnancies: A systematic review and meta-analysis. Obstetrics and Gynecology. 2013;**121**:1318-1326

[106] Hillman SC, Morris RK, Kilby MD. Co-twin prognosis after single fetal death: A systematic review and meta-analysis. Obstetrics and Gynecology. 2011;**118**:928-940

[107] Ong SS, Zamora J, Khan KS, Kilby MD. Prognosis for the co-twin following single-twin death: A systematic review. BJOG. 2006;**113**:992-998

[108] Karageyim Karsidag AY, Kars B, Dansuk R, Api O, Unal O, Turan MC, et al. Brain damage to the survivor within 30 min of co-twin demise in monochorionic twins. Fetal Diagnosis and Therapy. 2005;**20**:91-95

[109] Spong CY, Mercer BM, D'Alton M, Kilpatrick S, Blackwell S, Saade G. Timing of indicated late-preterm and early-term birth. Obstetrics and Gynecology. 2011;**118**:323-333

[110] Alexander GR, Kogan M, Martin J, Papiernik E. What are the fetal growth patterns of singletons, twins, and triplets in the United States? Clinical Obstetrics and Gynecology. 1998;**41**:114-125

[111] Giles W, Bisits A, O'Callaghan S, Gill A. The Doppler assessment in multiple pregnancy randomised controlled trial of ultrasound biometry versus umbilical artery Doppler ultrasound and biometry in twin pregnancy. DAMP Study Group. BJOG. 2003;**110**:593-597

[112] Twin-twin transfusion syndrome. Society for Maternal-Fetal Medicine [published erratum appears in Am J Obstet Gynecol 2013;208:392]. American Journal of Obstetrics and Gynecology. 2013;**208**:3-18

[113] Sueters M, Middeldorp JM, Lopriore E, Oepkes D, Kanhai HH, Vandenbussche FP. Timely diagnosis of twin-to-twin transfusion syndrome in monochorionic twin pregnancies by biweekly sonography combined with patient instruction to report onset of symptoms. Ultrasound in Obstetrics & Gynecology. 2006;**28**:659-664

[114] Royal College of Obstetricians and Gynaecologists. Consensus Views Arising from the 50th Study Group: Multiple Pregnancy. London: RCOG; 2006. Available from: http://www.rcog.org.uk/files/rcog-corp/uploaded-files/StudyGroupConsensusViews MultiplePregnancy.pdf [Accessed: 05 February 2014]

[115] Lewi L, Gucciardo L, Van Mieghem T, de Koninck P, Beck V, Medek H, et al. Monochorionic diamniotic twin pregnancies: Natural history and risk stratification. Fetal Diagnosis and Therapy. 2010;**27**:121-133

[116] Stamilio DM, Fraser WD, Moore TR. Twin-twin transfusion syndrome: An ethics-based and evidence-based argument for clinical research. American Journal of Obstetrics and Gynecology. 2010;**203**:3-16

[117] Slotnick RN, Ortega JE. Monoamniotic twinning and zona manipulation: A survey of U.S. IVF centers correlating zona manipulation procedures and high-risk twinning frequency. Journal of Assisted Reproduction and Genetics. 1996;**13**:381-385

[118] Baxi LV, Walsh CA. Monoamniotic twins in contemporary practice: A single-center study of perinatal outcomes. The Journal of Maternal-Fetal & Neonatal Medicine. 2010;**23**:506-510

[119] DeFalco LM, Sciscione AC, Megerian G, Tolosa J, Macones G, O'Shea A, et al. Inpatient versus outpatient management of monoamniotic twins and outcomes. American Journal of Perinatology. 2006;**23**:205-211

[120] Ezra Y, Shveiky D, Ophir E, Nadjari M, Eisenberg VH, Samueloff A, et al. Intensive management and early delivery reduce antenatal mortality in monoamniotic twin pregnancies. Acta Obstetricia et Gynecologica Scandinavica. 2005;**84**:432-435

[121] Sogaard K, Skibsted L, Brocks V. Acardiac twins: Pathophysiology, diagnosis, outcome and treatment. Six cases and review of the literature. Fetal Diagnosis and Therapy. 1999;**14**:53-59

[122] van Gemert MJ, Umur A, van den Wijngaard JP, VanBavel E, Vandenbussche FP, Nikkels PG. Increasing cardiac output and decreasing oxygenation sequence in pump twins of acardiac twin pregnancies. Physics in Medicine and Biology. 2005;**50**:N33-N42

[123] Mutchinick OM, Luna-Munoz L, Amar E, Bakker MK, Clementi M, Cocchi G, et al. Conjoined twins: A worldwide collaborative epidemiological study of the International Clearinghouse for Birth Defects Surveillance and Research. American Journal of Medical Genetics. Part C, Seminars in Medical Genetics. 2011;**157C**:274-287

[124] Spitz L, Kiely EM. Conjoined twins. JAMA. 2003;**289**:1307-1310

[125] Mackenzie TC, Crombleholme TM, Johnson MP, Schnaufer L, Flake AW, Hedrick HL, et al. The natural history of prenatally diagnosed conjoined twins. Journal of Pediatric Surgery. 2002;**37**:303-309

[126] Refuerzo JS, Momirova V, Peaceman AM, Sciscione A, Rouse DJ, Caritis SN, et al. Neonatal outcomes in twin pregnancies delivered moderately preterm, late preterm, and term. American Journal of Perinatology. 2010;**27**:537-542

[127] Cheung YB, Yip P, Karlberg J. Mortality of twins and singletons by gestational age: A varying-coefficient approach. American Journal of Epidemiology. 2000;**152**:1107-1116

[128] Crowther CA. Caesarean delivery for the second twin. Cochrane Database of Systematic Reviews. 2011;(12):CD000047. DOI: 10.1002/14651858.CD000047.pub2

[129] Barrett JF, Hannah ME, Hutton EK, Willan AR, Allen AC, Armson BA, et al. A randomized trial of planned cesarean or vaginal delivery for twin pregnancy. Twin Birth Study Collaborative Group [published erratum appears

in N Engl J Med 2013;369:2364]. The New England Journal of Medicine. 2013;**369**:1295-1305

[130] D'Alton ME. Delivery of the second twin: Revisiting the age-old dilemma. Obstetrics and Gynecology. 2010;**115**:221-222

[131] Grobman WA, Peaceman AM, Haney EI, Silver RK, MacGregor SN. Neonatal outcomes in triplet gestations after a trial of labor. American Journal of Obstetrics and Gynecology. 1998;**179**:942-945

[132] Alamia V Jr, Royek AB, Jaekle RK, Meyer BA. Preliminary experience with a prospective protocol for planned vaginal delivery of triplet gestations. American Journal of Obstetrics and Gynecology. 1998;**179**:1133-1135

[133] Wildschut HI, van Roosmalen J, van Leeuwen E, Keirse MJ. Planned abdominal compared with planned vaginal birth in triplet pregnancies. British Journal of Obstetrics and Gynaecology. 1995;**102**:292-296

[134] Sansregret A, Bujold E, Gauthier RJ. Twin delivery after a previous caesarean: A twelve-year experience. Journal of Obstetrics and Gynaecology Canada. 2003;**25**:294-298

[135] Cahill A, Stamilio DM, Pare E, Peipert JP, Stevens EJ, Nelson DB, et al. Vaginal birth after cesarean (VBAC) attempt in twin pregnancies: Is it safe? American Journal of Obstetrics and Gynecology. 2005;**193**:1050-1055

[136] Varner MW, Thom E, Spong CY, Landon MB, Leveno KJ, Rouse DJ, et al. Trial of labor after one previous cesarean delivery for multifetal gestation. National Institute of Child Health and Human Development (NICHD) Maternal-Fetal Medicine Units Network (MFMU). Obstetrics and Gynecology. 2007;**110**:814-819

[137] Myles T. Vaginal birth of twins after a previous Cesarean section. The Journal of Maternal-Fetal Medicine. 2001;**10**:171-174

[138] Miller DA, Mullin P, Hou D, Paul RH. Vaginal birth after cesarean section in twin gestation. American Journal of Obstetrics and Gynecology. 1996;**175**:194-198

[139] Francois K, Ortiz J, Harris C, Foley MR, Elliott JP. Is peripartum hysterectomy more common in multiple gestations? Obstetrics and Gynecology. 2005;**105**:1369-1372

[140] Quintero RA, Morales WJ, Allen MH, et al. Staging of twin-twin transfusion syndrome. Journal of Perinatology. 1999;**19**:550-555

Section 5

Case Report

Chapter 6

The Case of Langerhans Cell Histiocytosis (Abt-Letterer-Siwe Disease) in Twin Girls

Yakov Y. Yakovlev, Farok K. Manerov, Olga I. Andriyanova, Sergey A. Dudkin, Nataliya V. Matveeva, Nataliya V. Selivanova, Olga A. Zagorodnikova and Olga V. Domanskaya

Abstract

Abt-Letterer-Siwe disease is a form of Langerhans cell histiocytosis and occurs in 2–10 cases per 1 million of the child population per year. The Russian and foreign literature provide descriptions of this disease in children of different ages. Family cases of this pathology are described in a small number. The chapter presents a rare clinical observation of the Abt-Letterer-Siwe disease in twin girls.

Keywords: langerhans cell histiocytosis, Abt-Letterer-Siwe disease, children, twins, family case

1. Introduction

Langerhans cell histiocytosis (LCH) is a disease associated with abnormal proliferation and accumulation in the organs and tissues of pathological Langerhans cells, leading to local damage and violation of the affected organ function [1]. The term LCH includes eosinophilic granuloma, Hand-Schuller-Christian, and Abt-Letterer-Siwe diseases. The latter is considered the most difficult option with a mortality rate of at least 50% [2]. The study of Abt-Letterer-Siwe disease was started in 1924 by a German pathologist Erich Letterer [3]. In 1933, a Swedish pediatrician Sture Siwe published the first clinical description of the disease and proposed criteria for diagnosis [4]. In 1936, American authors Arthur Abt and Edward Denenholz in their publication proposed the adoption of the term "Letterer-Siwe disease" [5]. The disease is also mentioned in the literature as "Abt-Letterer-Siwe disease."

The LCH frequency is 2–10 cases per 1 million children in a year [1, 6–10]. Boys have this disease 1.5–2 times more often than girls, mainly in early childhood [1]. The skeleton (60–80%), skin (22–50%), lymph nodes (10–15%), liver (10–15%), bone marrow (10–15%), lungs (10–15%), endocrine glands (25%), central nervous system (2–4%), etc. [1, 11–13] may be involved in pathological process. These lesions are specific for Hand-Schuller-Christian and Abt-Letterer-Siwe diseases, but the latter is characterized by severity of the course, generalization of the process, and onset in the first years of life [7, 14, 15].

The involvement of skin in the process in 10% may be the only symptom [7, 13]. LCH foci on the skin are represented by yellowish-red, dense, highly itchy papules and nodules with a slight hemorrhagic hue, cracking is specific. Elements are localized in the retroauricular region, in large folds of the body. The scalp is affected like a seborrheic eczema type. With the development of the disease, the dissemination of rash occurs. For skin rash in case of LCH, a poor response to treatment with topical glucocorticosteroids is typical. In case of damage to the oral mucosa, ulcers with fibrinous plaque are formed [7]. The involvement of many organs and systems in the pathological process leads to the appearance of defects in the bones (mainly in flat bones), impaired hemostasis, lymphadenopathy, hepatosplenomegaly, and suppression of bone marrow function. Damage to the lungs is manifested by the spontaneous pneumothorax occurrence. Long, recurrent course of otitis is specific [1, 7, 14].

A probable clinical diagnosis is confirmed by histopathological and immunohistochemical methods. A biopsy of skin, osteolytic foci, and lymph nodes is preferred. Liver or lung biopsy is performed in the absence of other materials [1]. Light microscopy does not allow an unambiguous diagnosis. The "gold standard" of diagnosis is the identification of Birbeck granules by electron microscopy. A more sensitive and specific diagnostics is immunohistochemical staining with langerin (CD 207), which is a monoclonal antibody against type II transmembrane protein bound to the Birbeck granules [13].

According to the data of Moskacheva et al., until 1931, about 65 cases of Hand-Schuller-Christian disease and 4 cases of Abt-Letterer-Siwe disease were described. According to other authors to 1955 described about 350 and 68 cases of the disease it [15]. In the Russian Scientific Electronic Library in the period from 2004 till 2017, about 8 clinical observations of this disease in children were described. PubMed's English language text database for the same period represents more than 300 sources, including cases of Abt-Letterer-Siwe.

Until the middle of the twentieth century, the relationship of Abt-Letterer-Siwe disease with genetic disorders was questioned [5, 15]. The described family cases in siblings and, moreover, cases of the disease in twins were of particular interest. The Russian language descriptive works of the LCH family cases, including the disease Abt-Letterer-Siwe, in the Russian Scientific Electronic Library for the last 10–15 years are absent. Over the past 50–60 years, we have found about 40 LCH familial cases (half of Abt-Letterer-Siwe disease) in the PubMed database, of which 12 are twins with a description of the disease.

Due to the pathology rarity, we represent a description of the Abt-Letterer-Siwe disease case in two monozygotic twin girls A and E, who were admitted to our clinic at the age of 12 months.

2. Description of the Abt-Letterer-Siwe disease case

Children are from monozygotic twins from one pregnancy. Parents are young and healthy. Delivery occurred at a period of 34 weeks. Both children were switched to artificial feeding during the first month. The development of children throughout the observation period corresponded to the age.

For the first time, parents noted the appearance of moderately itchy skin rash and ulcerative stomatitis in children at the age of 1.5–2 months. Hyperemia, papules, crusts were present in the area of large skin folds (cervical, axillary, inguinal). The boundaries of skin changes were legibly delineated (**Figure 1**). Quickly enough, the scalp (hyperemia, severe desquamation, yellowish crusts, papules) and the parotid area (hyperemia, crusts, papules, weeping) were involved in the process. Rare small

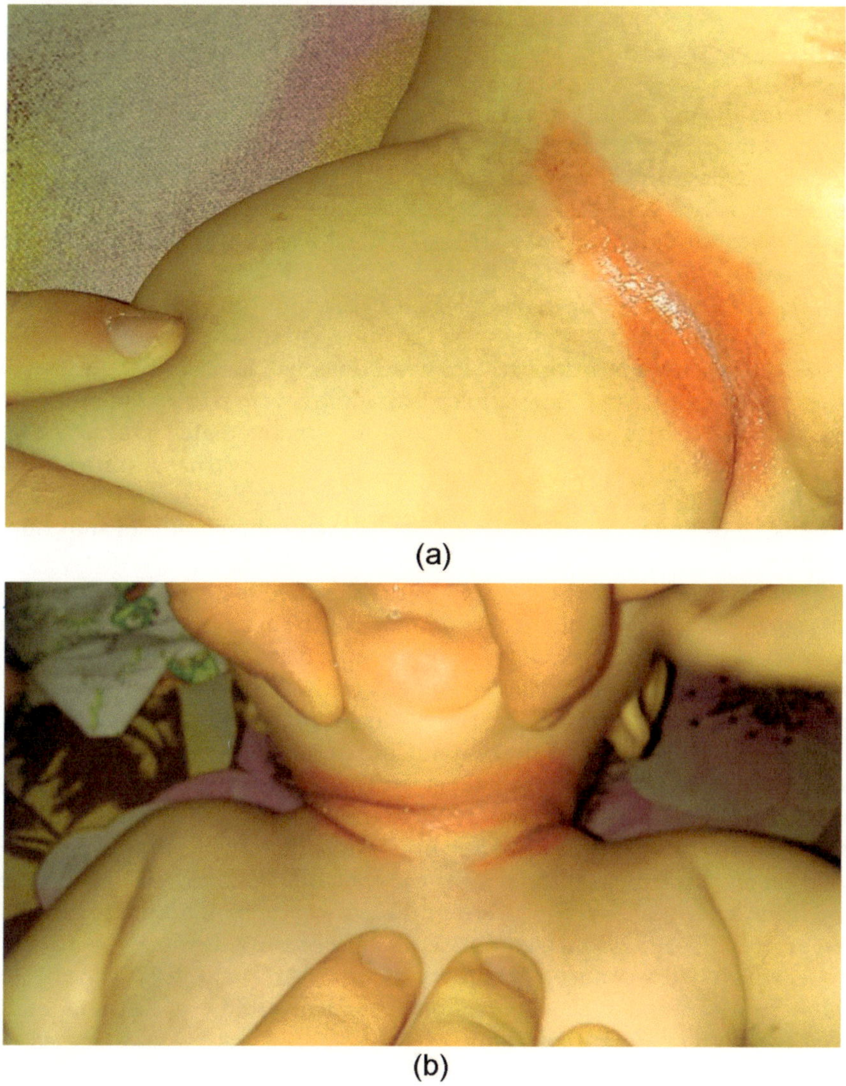

Figure 1.
Skin changes: inguinal fold (a) and neck fold (b).

papules and pustules occasionally appeared on the skin of the limbs and trunk (outside the folds), which was considered as pyodermia. Secondary changes, such as small scars, remained in place of some papules and pustules. In a retrospective assessment, it is possible that there were small nodules on the skin. Children received antihistamines, care cosmetics, and topical corticosteroids; milk mixtures were changed. No improvement was observed. The application of topical corticosteroids to the affected areas exacerbated itching and hyperemia, and anxiety appeared in children.

Over the next 4–5 months, against the background of the treatment variety, skin manifestations persisted in a stable condition of children and sufficient weight gain. On the scalp ("seborrheic area") and the parotid region, yellowish crusts, erythema, peeling, papules, and weeping were observed.

The main changes were localized in large folds, which were manifested by hyperemia, papules, crusts, and cracks. Soles, palms, and interdigital spaces were involved in the process, where hyperemia, peeling, yellowish crusts, and cracks were observed. The skin of the limbs, trunk, and face was intact, with the exception of rare episodes of pustular rash. Despite extensive and persistent skin lesions, itching was moderate. During the periods of exacerbation, children became restless due to pain.

The dermatologist examined the children at the age of 7 months for the first time. Bright erythema-squamous rash with weeping and mucous discharge in the area of large folds were described, scars after previous pustulosis. Erythematous diaper rash and atopic dermatitis were diagnosed. Antihistamines, topical glucocorticoids, and antibiotics were administered as treatment. After 2 weeks, no significant dynamics were observed.

At the age of 9 months, the dermatologists in the clinic diagnosed an infant form of atopic dermatitis. Skin symptoms were the same. On the part of the internal organs and in blood tests, no significant pathology was detected. In bacteriological studies from the inguinal, axillary, and neck folds, *Staphylococcus aureus* was identified. Girls received a dairy-free diet, a solution of potassium permanganate on the affected skin folds, nystatin, hydrocortisone + oxytetracycline, and papaverine ointment. Children were discharged without improvement at the age of 9 months 3 weeks with recommendations for treatment of intestinal dysbiosis, a hypoallergenic diet and continued local therapy.

At the age of 11 months, the children were examined by a pediatrician in the consultation center. During physical examination, the attention was paid to the course of the disease, which was atypical for atopic dermatitis—localization of rash was mainly in skin folds of the "diaper dermatitis" type of dark-red color with a relatively intact remaining surface, damage of the palms, soles, interdigital spaces of the feet, ulceration of the oral mucosa in the onset, episodes of pustular rash with an outcome in small scars, repeated worsening of symptoms (increased hyperemia, increased itching, and the appearance of pain) when using topical glucocorticosteroids, the absence of any improvement after the exclusion of cow's milk protein from the diet (at the time of the consultation, the children received a high-hydrolysis formula for a long time and scanty complementary foods). The girls showed periodic weeping in the ears area, damage of the entire scalp like a seborrhea type, which had an unusually stubborn course. An anamnesis of the disease, clinical picture, absence of the effect of glucocorticosteroids, and a therapeutic diet excluded the atopic dermatitis diagnosis.

At the age of 12 months, the condition worsened and the children were admitted to our clinic. Children had fever up to 39–40°C, intoxication, and moderate hepatosplenomegaly. Skin symptoms significantly increased (**Figure 2**). In the clinical blood analysis of girls A and E, anemia (erythrocytes 3.32 and $3.58*10^{12}$/L, and hemoglobin 75 and 84 g/L, respectively), leukocytes at level $5.8*10^{9}$/L and $9.3*10^{9}$/L, respectively, thrombocytopenia (platelets 66 and $108*10^{9}$/L, respectively), and ESR 20 mm/h in both girls were observed. The range of differential diagnosis included primary immunodeficiency, psoriasis, and LCH. During one day, the children received intravenous immunoglobulin based on the course dose of 1 g/kg due to the severity of the condition and a probable diagnosis of immunodeficiency.

The condition of children remained serious due to an increase in hematological disorders (anemia—hemoglobin up to 70–90 g/L, thrombocytopenia up to single cells, and leukopenia up to 3–4 M09/L), hemorrhagic (bleeding of elements in large-folds) and hepatolienal syndromes, fever up to 39–40°C, and infection of the skin—primarily with "wild," and then with hospital strains of bacteria. An intensive, replacement therapy and an antibiotic therapy were applied.

During treatment, a temporary improvement was observed in the form of drying, reduction of purulent crusts, and improvement of well-being. On the 10th day of hospitalization, child A developed a septic shock. In the intensive care unit,

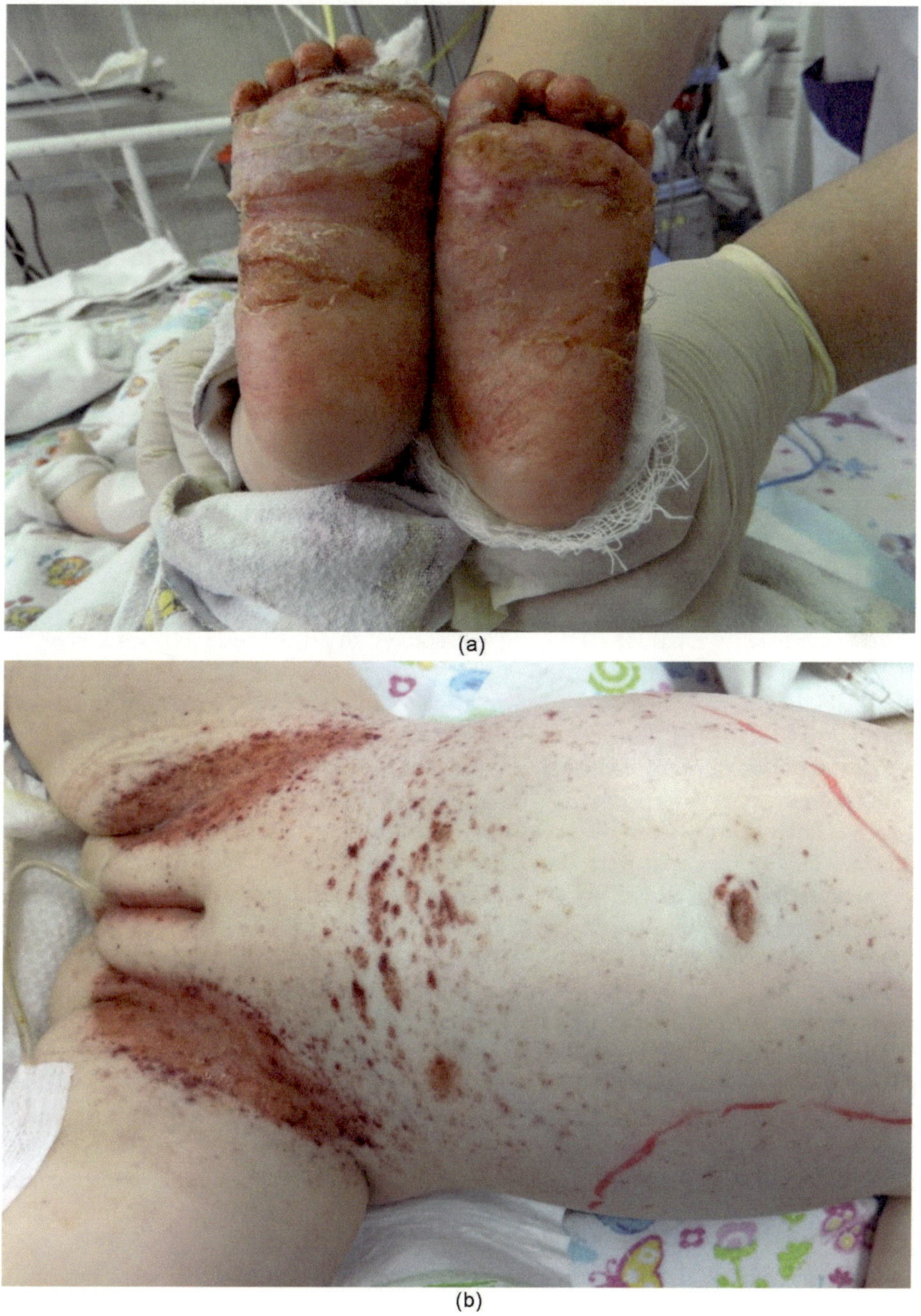

Figure 2.
Dynamics of skin changes: foot skin lesion (a) and inguinal areas (b).

the girl was on the mechanical ventilation of lungs for 10 days. The condition of the second child remained stably severe.

Both girls excluded HIV infection, primary immunodeficiencies of the humoral, cellular, and phagocytic parts of the immune system, and violation of complement. Specific lesions of bones and lungs were excluded according to X-ray and computed tomography (CT) results. In child E, according to spiral CT, a left-sided otitis media was observed without destructive changes. According to bone marrow puncture, in child A, the process disorders differentiation and the maturation of cells were not determined, the erythroid germ was expanded, and a moderate delay in maturation at the level of myelocytes was observed in the granulocytic germ. Megakaryocytes were not found during the study. Free platelets were isolated.

In a cytological study of smear impressions from the creases in child A, in addition to inflammatory elements and eosinophils, cells with hyperchromic sharply enlarged nuclei, with signs of nuclear polymorphism and atypia, and binuclear cells were found. Atypical large cells with an oval nucleus, fine-grained chromatin, containing 1–2 nucleoli, and an abundant pale-stained cytoplasm were visualized in a significant amount. Some cells contained vacuoles.

The child A underwent a skin biopsy from a pathological focus. Light microscopy in the papillary layer at the border with the epidermis revealed single foci of proliferation of large oval and process cells with an eosinophilic cytoplasm, hyperchromic nuclei, and single binuclear cells. The described that the morphology was specific for histiocytosis. In the Federal State Budgetary Institution "National Medical Research Center named after Dmitry Rogachev" (Moscow), an immunohistochemical study was performed. According to this analysis, large cells express Langerin, CD13, and single cells express CD68. Reactions with other antibodies to them are negative. Conclusion: LCH.

Two weeks after admission to the hospital, an intravenous administration of glucocorticosteroids at a dose 20 mg/kg was started in pulse mode 3 times a week with further switch to oral administration of prednisolone at a dose 2 mg/kg. Confirmation of the LCH diagnosis (Abt-Letterer-Siwe disease) made it possible to continue therapy according to the LCH III protocol in the Pediatric Oncohematology Department. Against the background of some stabilization of the condition, episodes of fever, hepatosplenomegaly, pancytopenia in the clinical blood analysis, and bleeding persisted. Rash in large skin folds was without significant dynamics. Taking it into account, a lack of response to therapy was reported. Children were directed to the Federal State Budgetary Institution "National Medical Research Center named after Dmitry Rogachev" (Moscow) for further treatment.

Our clinical case of Abt-Letterer-Siwe disease is one of the most severe LCH variants. In children, there was a multisystem lesion, involving the liver, hematopoietic system, and spleen, which is prognostically unfavorable. A feature of the described case is the simultaneous onset of the disease in two twin girls, which is an extremely rare observation. This clinical case shows the difficulty in diagnosing LCH (Abt-Letterer-Siwe disease) at an early age. Difficulties in making a diagnosis arise when there is still no developed clinical symptomatology of the disease or the clinical picture is inapparent [15]. The prevalence of damage to one organ or system, especially at the beginning of the disease, leads to erroneous diagnoses. In our clinical case, the main symptom of the disease during 10–11 months in both girls was skin damage. During this period of time, they were observed by pediatricians and dermatologists with a diagnosis of atopic dermatitis and diaper rash.

3. Conclusions

In our opinion, the attending physician should have been alerted by a number of symptoms that are not specific for atopic dermatitis: ulcerative stomatitis in the onset; absolutely unspecific localization of the rash—large folds without damage to the skin areas typical for atopic dermatitis at this age; unusual coloring of elements (dark-red); damage of the palms, soles, and interdigital spaces; episodes of an abscess rash that left small scars—this symptom indicates a deeper lesion of the skin than with ordinary pyodermia; and one of the significant symptoms is the deterioration of skin symptoms with the "gold standard" topical application treatment of atopic dermatitis—topical glucocorticosteroids. The latter manifestation is typical for the Abt-Letterer-Siwe disease, but is absolutely not specific for allergic rash.

Thus, at present, the diagnosis of orphan diseases remains difficult at the early stages. This is due to the polymorphism of manifestations, the rarity of cases, and the similarity with other nosologies.

Conflict of interest

The authors of the chapter confirmed the absence of financial support for the study that needs to be reported and declare no conflict of interest.

Author details

Yakov Y. Yakovlev[1*], Farok K. Manerov[1], Olga I. Andriyanova[2], Sergey A. Dudkin[3], Nataliya V. Matveeva[4], Nataliya V. Selivanova[3], Olga A. Zagorodnikova[1] and Olga V. Domanskaya[5]

1 Pediatrics and Neonatology Department, Novokuznetsk State Institute of Postgraduate Medicine, Russian Medical Academy of Continuous Professional Education, The Ministry of Health of Russian Federation, Novokuznetsk, Russia

2 Department of Reanimation and Anesthesiology, Novokuznetsk City Children's Clinical Hospital No. 4, Novokuznetsk, Russia

3 Department of Pediatric Oncology and Hematology, Novokuznetsk City Children's Clinical Hospital No. 4, Novokuznetsk, Russia

4 Department of Pediatrics, Novokuznetsk City Children's Clinical Hospital No. 4, Novokuznetsk, Russia

5 Novokuznetsk City Children's Clinical Hospital No. 4, Novokuznetsk, Russia

*Address all correspondence to: yko3@yandex.ru

References

[1] Rumyantsev AG, Maschan AA, Maschan MA, Novichkova GA. Federal clinical guidelines for the diagnosis and treatment of histiocytosis from Langerhans cells in children. Moscow; 2015. pp. 1-39 (in Russian)

[2] Yusupova LA, Yunusova EI, Garayeva ZS, Mavlyutova GI. Histiocyitosis X. Practical Medicine. 2014;**8**(84):7-10

[3] Letterer E. Aleukamische Retikulose. (Ein Beitrag zu den proliferativen Erkrankungen des Retikuloendothelialen apparates). Frankfurter Zeitschrift für Pathologie. 1924;**30**:377-394

[4] Siwe SA. Die Reiticuloendotheliose — ein neues Krankheitsbild unter den Hepatosphlenomegalien. Z. Kinder-Heilk. 1933;**55**:212-247. DOI: 10.1007/BF02251373

[5] Abt AF, Denenholz EJ. Letterer-Siwe's disease: Spleno-hepatomegaly associated with wide-spread hyperplasia of nonlipoid-storing macrophages; discussion of the so-called reticulo-endothelioses. American Journal of Diseases of Children. 1936;**51**(3):499-522

[6] Odinets Yu V, Poddubnaya IN, Makeeva NI. Histiocytosis from Langerhans cells in children. Child Health. 2016;**4**(72):89-91

[7] Heger PG. In: Kubanova AA, Lvov AN, editors. Pediatric Dermatology: Translation from German. Moscow: Panfilov Publishing House, BINOM. Knowledge Laboratory; 2013. pp. 476-482

[8] Arico M, Nichols K, Whitlock JA, Arceci R, Haupt R, Mittler U, et al. Familial clustering of Langerhans cell histiocytosis. British Journal of Haematology. 1999;**107**(4):883-888

[9] Minkov M. Multisystem Langerhans cell histiocytosis in children: Current treatment and future directions. Paediatric Drugs. 2011;**13**(2):75-86

[10] Morren M-A, Broecke KV, Vangeebergen L, Sillevis-Smitt JH, Van Den Berghe P, Hauben E, et al. Diverse cutaneous presentations of Langerhans cell histiocytosis in children: A retrospective cohort study. Pediatric Blood & Cancer. 2016;**63**(3):486-492

[11] Emile J-F, Abla O, Fraitag S, Horne A, Haroche J, Donadieu J, et al. Revised classification of histiocytoses and neoplasms of the macrophage-dendritic cell lineages. Blood. 2016;**127**(22):2672-2681

[12] Haupt R, Minkov M, Astigarraga I, Schafer E, Nanduri V, Jubran R, et al. Langerhans cell histiocytosis (LCH): Guidelines for diagnosis, clinical workup, and treatment for patients till the age of 18 years. Pediatric Blood & Cancer. 2013;**60**(2):175-184

[13] Satter EK, High WA. Langerhans cell histiocytosis: A review of the current recommendations of the Histiocyte Society. Pediatric Dermatology. 2008;**25**(3):291-295

[14] Glushkov AV, Andriyanova OI, Manerov FK, Yu MY, Loktionov AA. Histiocytosis from Langerhans cells with isolated lung damage in a child of three years. General Resuscitation. 2009;**5**(2):66-69

[15] Moskacheva KA, Nebolsin LI, Znamenskaya IV. Reticulohistiocytosis in Children. Medicina: Leningrad; 1967